AUTHENTIC
INDIAN HEAD MASSAGE
'MALISH'

AUTHENTIC
INDIAN HEAD MASSAGE
'MALISH'

Kush Kumar

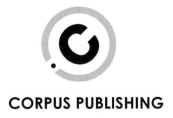

CORPUS PUBLISHING

First published in 2002 by
Corpus Publishing Limited
4/5 The Marina, Harbour Road, Lydney, Gloucestershire, GL15 5ET

Disclaimer
This publication is intended as an informational guide. The techniques described are a supplement and not a substitute for professional tuition. Whilst the information herein is supplied in good faith, no responsibility is taken by either the publisher or the author for any damage, injury or loss, however caused, which may arise from the use of the information provided.

Acknowledgements
I would like to thank all of those who participated in making this book possible. Also, the research and depth of knowledge of those who saw a need to educate for the purpose of bringing intuitive knowledge to the conscious mind. Dr. P. Kulkarni, Jolanta Basnyet, Russell King, Marina and Tony Wilson, Roseline Bourt, Peter Mason, my niece and nephew Gino and Bonice Masih, my sister Asha Rani, Robert Ruddock and to my very special friend, Naomi Mehta, for her sound advice and inspiration in completing this project. Due acknowledgement is given to the book by Su Fox and Damien Pritchard, 'Anatomy, Physiology and Pathology for the Massage Therapist', which forms the basis of Part 3.

British Library Cataloguing in Publication Data
A CIP record for this book is available from the British Library
ISBN 1 903333 14 8

Text and Cover Design Rob Benson
Photography David Oldridge
Anatomical Drawings Amanda Williams
Printed and bound in Hong Kong through Printworks International Ltd.

Contents

Dedication

This book has been written in memory of my grandfather based upon his values and teachings. At a very young age, he began to teach me about my own personal journey into life and how to overcome various hurdles, with his continuous efforts and motivation. I have been able to realise a wish and contribute a method of therapy to guide people towards a more meaningful life.

This book maps out a personal opinion of the therapy and enlists experiences shared. It is based on lifelong learning of the East and the West and is authentic to my own values and experiences. With the help of friends and active professionals in society, this book has been made possible.

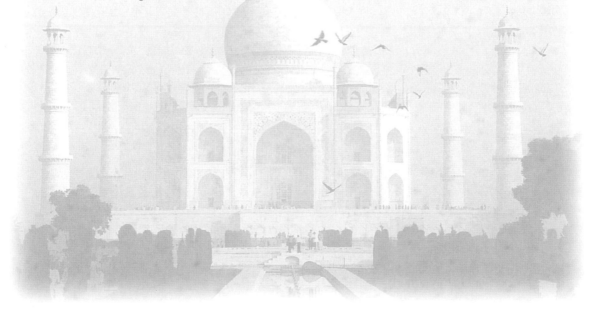

Part I
An Introduction to Indian Head Massage

The Indian head, neck, shoulder, face and ear massage is becoming increasingly popular and sought after in the West. Colleges and therapy centres now regularly feature the treatment along with more established complementary therapies. The aim of this textbook is to guide the many therapists and student therapists through both the practical and theoretical aspects of Indian Head Massage, providing both Eastern and Western approaches to the treatment.

The book can be used as a comprehensive reference for students wishing to practice the therapy. The author is a qualified lecturer and authority on Indian Head Massage.

In addition, the text is intended as a support to various examining boards currently available in local and national training institutes for Indian Head Massage. In particular, the book covers core syllabus material in the CAT (Confederation of Ayurvedic Therapy) Diplomas which are regulated by The Confederation of Indian Head Massage, VTCT and Edexcel B/Tec. Other examining and awarding bodies will inevitably expand into this field, and the text will be sufficiently comprehensive to support any future syllabus on the subject.

The Principles of Ayurveda/healing

Ayurveda, the science of life, is undoubtedly the oldest medical system recorded. It is based on a fundamental understanding of human existence. According to the ancient Ayurvedic beliefs, mortal man exists on three levels; through his mind, his physical body and his life force or spirit.

There are three respective needs. Firstly, that of the mind (healing of mental or psychological disorders) such as fear, anger, bad habits and the lack of both initiative and confidence. The second is that of the body, to be free of physical suffering and to control physical disorders and disease. The third, which is frequently ignored or sometimes not even recognised in the West, is that of the spirit or soul.

Spiritual disorders manifest themselves as indifference, lack of purpose, contentment with the material side of existence and ignorance of the laws of life and of man's own divinity. The attention of most people is fixed solely on the cure of bodily disharmony because it is so tangible and obvious. They do not realise that their mental disturbances of worry and egotism and their spiritual blindness to the divine meaning of life are the real causes of all human misery. It is only when man destroys the mental blockages of intolerance, rage, fear and has freed his soul from ignorance, that he will cease to suffer from physical or mental disease.

Some physicians of ancient India, working under the influence of the Lord Buddha, advanced the art of healing to so perfect a state that they were able to abolish surgery, even though the surgery of that time was as efficient, or more so, than that of the present day. Modern medical science often deals with the result and not the causes of disharmony.

In the East, since ancient times, the body has been thought of as a 'Shrine of the Spirit' where the power of nature dwelled. However, in modern times the influence of science in modern medicine has reduced the professional healing system to focussing on the body without proper sensitivity to the 'whole person' described in ancient medical texts. Only now are we beginning to realise the accuracy of that philosophy and to promote the concept of holistic (whole) therapy. Rational thought, which relies on the function of the forebrain, suppresses the function of the midbrain, which is responsible for our emotion and instincts.

When the activity is suppressed here, it becomes difficult for people to express themselves and to experience life fully. It is only when the true state of illness is diagnosed from the point of view of the holistic nature of life and of the interrelationship of the whole being rather than on physical symptoms, that a true cure can be affected.

Ayurveda, the ancient Indian system of medicine, can be literally translated into English; it is composed of two words, *Ayu* and *Veda*. Ayu means life and Veda denotes the science, i.e. science of life. Ayu is defined as a combination of *Sharira* (body), *Indriya* (senses), *Mana* (mind) and *Atma* (spirit/soul). Body without senses, mind and spirit/soul is dead and it is not Ayu. In the West, health has only recently begun to be defined by the World Health Organisation in terms not only of the absence of physical disease but also in terms of positive mental state and general feelings of wellbeing. The current health manifesto from most Western governments accepts that mental illness is a major cause of death in developed countries and there is now a move towards promoting health from a more holistic medical approach.

Therefore, while defining health (*Swastha*), it has long been recognised by the ancient system that a person having equilibrium of *Dosha* and *Agni* (digestive and metabolic enzymes) with proper functioning of *Dhatu* (tissues) and *Mala* (metabolic by-products and excretions), who also possesses happiness and balance of *Atma* (spirit/soul), *Indriya* (senses) and *Mana* (mind), has attained Swastha or good health. Thus, Ayurveda deals with the diseased person and not solely with the disease. It is an ancient holistic approach which, centuries later, is finding favour amongst those concerned with the health of individuals and populations.

Ayurveda has three main aims. To:

1.   Promote the health of the healthy persons.
2.   Preserve the health.
3.   Cure or control the disease of the patient.

It fulfils these aims through eight branches:

1.   Kayachikitsa (internal medicine).
2.   Shalya Tantra (surgery).
3.   Shalakya Tantra (otorhinolaryngology (ENT) and ophthalmology).
4.   Kaumara Bhrutya (paediatric and obstetric).

5.   Rasayana (rejuvenation).
6.   Vajikarana (aphrodisiac).
7.   Agada Tantra (toxicology), and;
8.   Bhuta Vidya (psychotherapy).

Out of these, generally Rasayana and Vajikarana, including *Swasthavrutta*, deal with the preservation and promotion of the health of the healthy persons and the remaining branches deal with the diseased person.

Pancha Mahabhuta – The Five Universal Elements

From the Indian philosophical point of view, all the matters of the universe are made up of five elements, collectively known as Pancha Mahabhuta (five basic elements). These are Aakasha (space), Vayu (air), Agni (fire), Jala (water), and Pruthvi (earth). Each of these can be perceived by its distinctive quality: Aakasha by Shabda (sound), Vayu by Sparsha (touch), Agni by Rupa (colour), Jala by Rasa (taste), and Pruthvi by Gandha (odour, smell).

Purusha

The body is termed Purusha when Atma (soul) joins with Pancha Mahabhuta (five basic elements) and then matter assumes life. In Ayurveda, the term Purusha is specifically used for human beings. Thus, Pancha Mahabhuta are the basic elements required for the formation of all the bodily tissues, sensory and motor organs, and mind.

Dosha

The concept of Dosha has been evolved by the great sages of Ayurveda, to *differentiate between living and non-living entities*. Though Sharira (human body) is made up of Pancha Mahabhuta, it attains life only when Atma (soul), Indriya (senses) and Mana (mind) join to it. Dosha are the biological units of the living body which are responsible for all its functions. There are three distinct Dosha: Vata, Pitta and Kapha. Each Dosha is made up from different elements of the five universal elements already identified.

•   Vata is formed from Vayu (air) and Akasha (space).
•   Pitta is formed from Agni (fire).
•   Kapha is formed from Pruthvi (earth) and Jala (water).

In the normal state of equilibrium, the Dosha support the body and its functions but when the balance of the elements within the individual Dosha are disturbed, the Dosha itself can produce symptoms of disease. Thus, Dosha plays an important role in the pathogenesis, diagnosis and treatment of any disease.

Vata

The word '*Vata*' is derived from the verb 'Va', which means 'Gati' (*to move*). This Dosha is responsible for all the movements in the body which can be broken down to cover five areas:

1. *Prana Vayu*. The seat of function of *Prana Vayu* is: i. head, ii. chest, iii. throat, iv. tongue, v. mouth, and vi. nose. It controls the functions of: i. salivation, ii. eructation (belching), iii. sneezing, and iv. respiration.

2. *Udana Vayu*. The seat of function of *Udana Vayu* is: i. umbilicus, ii. chest, and iii. throat. Its main function is sound production (phonation). It also provides: i. enthusiasm, ii. vitality, and iii. complexion to human beings.

3. *Samana Vayu*. Functions of *Samana Vayu* are closely related to Agni (digestive juices = fire). It: i. regulates the secretion of the gastric juice, ii. retains the food in the stomach or intestine for the required time, and iii. thus helps in its absorption.

4. *Vyana Vayu,* which is situated all over the body, is responsible for: i. pulsation of the heart, ii. blood circulation, and iii. controlling the movement of eyes and limbs.

5. *Apana Vayu*. The seat of function of *Apana Vayu* is: i. testes, ii. bladder, iii. umbilical region, iv. thigh, and v. groin. It controls the elimination of: i. semen, ii. urine, and iii. faeces. Apana Vayu also governs the movements related with the delivery of foetus.

Pitta

The word '*Pitta*' is derived from the root 'Tapa', which means 'Santapa' (heat). This Dosha is responsible for digestion and metabolism of the body. It consists of five types:

1.   *Pachaka Pitta* is located in the Grahani (stomach and intestine). Its main functions are digestion, and to augment the other Pitta situated in the body.
2.   *Ranjaka Pitta* are liver and spleen. Its main function is to convert Rasa (plasma fluid) into Rakta (blood).
3.   *Bhrajaka Pitta* is found in the skin and provides pigment to the skin and hair.
4.   *Alochaka Pitta* is situated in the eye, and its functions are vision and discrimination of colours.
5.   *Sadhaka Pitta* is located in the Hrudaya (heart) and it is responsible for intelligence and ego. It is due to this Pitta that all the functions of the mind and the body are co-ordinated.

Kapha

Kapha is also called Shleshma. One of its main functions is to provide nutrition to the bodily tissues. Kapha also consists of five types:

1.   *Kledaka Kapha* is situated in the stomach. It is slimy and sticky (Pichila) in quality, sweet in taste and has the action of moistening the food ingested. It also protects the digestive organs from being hurt by the digestive juices.
2.   *Avalambaka Kapha* is located in the chest where it provides the nutrition to the heart.
3.   *Bodhaka Kapha* is found in the tongue and it is responsible for perceiving the taste.
4.   The seat of function of *Shleshaka Kapha* is the joints where it provides lubrication to allow the joints to function properly.
5.   *Tarpaka Kapha* is situated in the head and gives nutrition to the mental faculties.

Manas Dosha

In addition to Vata, Pitta and Kapha which are the bodily Dosha, there are two Manas Dosha: Rajas (passion) and Tamas (darkness). Manas Dosha may be held responsible for mental diseases.

Dushya – Disease

In the disease process, Dosha are initially vitiated (debased), which renders the Dhatu and Mala (*see* below) inefficient in their functions. As Dhatu and Mala get vitiated by Dosha, they are also named as Dushya. In the normal condition, Dosha, Dhatu and Mala support the body, but when vitiated, produce the disease.

Dhatu

The word *'Dhatu'* is derived from the verb 'Dha', which means to 'hold'. The matters which hold the body, are termed as Dhatu. In general, it incorporates the following seven types:

1.   Rasa (nourishing fluid of plasma).
2.   Rakta (blood).
3.   Mamsa (muscular tissue).
4.   Meda (fatty tissue).
5.   Asthi (bone and connective tissues).
6.   Majja (bone marrow).
7.   Shukra (vital substance).

There are three types of pathological changes in these Dhatu:

1.   Kshaya (decrease).
2.   Vruddhi (increase), and;
3.   Pradosha (vitiation or disabling).

The Kshaya of the one and the Vruddhi of the other, may be simultaneous in the same disease and in the same patient. In this condition, the Dhatu increases at one place at the cost of the other.

Upadhatu

The Upadhatu are generally less prone to taking part in the early disease process but can nevertheless be vitiated by Dosha. They are often found playing a supporting role to the Dhatu and include:

1.   Stanya (breast milk).
2.   Artava (menstrual blood).
3.   Kandara (tendons).
4.   Shira (vessels).
5.   Vasa (fat).
6.   Twak (skin).
7.   Snayu (muscle).

Mala

Mala are different excretions which can be adversely affected by Dhosa imbalances and are often seen as an initial symptom of disease or Dushya where abnormal excretion patterns are observed.

1. Faeces – diarrhoea or constipation are both indications of Dhosa imbalances but also the colour of the faeces may indicate more specific disease.
2. Urine – frequent urination is often found to be an early symptom of diabetes and the colour and smell of the urine can also indicate high levels of sugar or protein excretion or even dehydration.
3. Mala Kapha – lubricants for joint mobility, digestion and protection from acid attack of internal tissues.
4. Mala Pitta – digestive enzyme excretions and natural oils for protection of skin and hair.
5. Sweda (sweat).
6. Nakha (nails).

Srotas

The word 'Srotas' is derived from 'Sru', which means 'oozing'. The oozing of nourishing fluid and the return of waste matters take place through these Srotas. In fact, the whole body is composed of Srotas, but for the convenience of diagnosis and treatment, they have been classified into thirteen groups. They are:

1. Prana-Vaha (channels through which oxygen and carbon dioxide exchange takes place).
2. Udaka-Vaha (water balance).
3. Anna-Vaha (food passage).
4. Rasa-Vaha (plasma movement).
5. Rakta-Vaha (blood circulation).
6. Mamsa-Vaha (muscular tissue).
7. Meda-Vaha (fat).
8. Asthi-Vaha (connective tissue).
9. Majja-Vaha (bone marrow).
10. Shukra-Vaha (semen).
11. Mutra-Vaha (urinary channels).
12. Purisha-Vaha (channel for faeces).
13. Sweda-Vaha (channel for sweat).

The pathological conditions in these Srotas are:

1.   Atipravutti (excessive flow).
2.   Sangraha (accumulation).
3.   Vimarga-Gamana (leakage/haemorrhage).
4.   Sira-Granthi (thrombosis).

Any one, two, three or even four types of pathological conditions may occur in the disease.

Agni

Agni is a very important factor because Ayurveda believes that the majority, if not all the diseases are caused by an imbalance of Agni. It is responsible for all the digestion and metabolism of the body. It has thirteen functions which are potential targets for disturbance, but of these, Jatharagni (digestive enzymes and juices) are the most important, with all others being dependent on it. The vitiation of these Agni are of three types:

1.   Vishmagni, (irregular).
2.   Tikshagni (extensive), and;
3.   Mandagni (low).

These three abnormalities of Agni are responsible for producing various types of disease, but Mandagni is the most common cause of disease.

Ayurvedic Healing

Healing is a natural power in man. The healing of others is possible through willpower which is uninterrupted by the lower mind or conscious thought. The therapist's attitude of mind constitutes a vital element in the art of massage. Techniques are used to voluntarily withdraw the mind from the senses and focus inwardly to reveal the centre of consciousness. A mind with one focus creates a dynamic will, which can be used for healing. The therapist needs to be highly sensitive and aware and must not impose ideas, techniques or solutions on the body to rectify a problem or mask symptoms. They must try to awaken the native intelligence of the body.

General Information on Indian Head Massage

The art of Indian Head Massage is an Ayurvedic form of healing and relaxation which is used widely in Asia, mainly by masseurs and hairdressers, to combat daily tensions and stress. The technique has been passed down families for several generations and brings immediate relief and relaxation on a deeper level than is possible with other massage techniques. However, many years and even centuries ago, when men and woman kept longer hair, the bonding communication of massage was applied in the home.

Therapies for relaxation, especially in the Western commercial marketplace will inevitably focus on the benefits for the recipient being the person who pays cash for the privilege. However, that is denying a vital aspect of the Ayurvedic healing process. As stated earlier, healing is a natural power in man, and such power is often ignored. Ayurvedic massage should also offer an individual the power to explore and develop their inner healing potential and through this become empowered to ensure their own wellbeing as well as that of others. Awareness of recent trends in medicine show that modern physicians have begun to deal with subtle forms of energy in both the diagnosis and treatment of illness, correspondingly subtler approaches in therapy are required with principles and interventions involving the mind, body and spiritual dimensions.

An Indian Head Massage soothes, comforts and harmonises the body's natural balance, helping to promote physical and psychological wellbeing, which will leave the client with a sense of focus, clarity and vision. It incorporates the laying on of hands, thumb and finger pressure, effleurage and friction movements.

Acupressure points are stimulated, which improves the circulation of the blood and lymphatic fluid and the broader physical techniques reduce muscular and nervous tension. The cells are provided with an opportunity for optimal oxygenation, and the improved circulation stimulates a faster flow and excretion of both physical and emotional toxins. The tissues of the neck and shoulders are stretched and mobilised. A stiff neck can be caused by anything from stress or sitting in a draught, to sleeping in an uncomfortable position or watching too many games of tennis. However, it is one of the simplest ailments to cure with a lot of simple movements and plenty of warming repetitions, plus some kneading strokes to relax and release any areas with trapped nerves or muscle tension.

There is a thin layer of muscle covering the skull which tightens when we are tense, causing headaches and a feeling of anxiety. Since the scalp retains a lot of tension, massage can be used to relax this area and tone the muscles to prevent future tightening under stress, thus helping not only to relieve immediate complaints but also to actively prevent any further reoccurence. Remember that the Ayurvedic system is concerned with not only the cure and control but also the promotion and prevention of disease. The head massage can also be used to relieve eyestrain and eye tension and can often provide immediate results in terms of colour perception with many recipients of the massage being able to see colours more vividly.

Vascular headaches including migraines as well as psychogenic headaches (caused by tension, anxiety and depression) can often be relieved by this form of massage since the treatment not only deals with the physical causes but also can incorporate an holistic approach to the healing, taking into account the more emotional and psychological factors involved.

The clinical explanation for the experience of headache is that blood vessels in the head increase in size. As these arteries are usually accompanied by nerves, when enlarged, they press on the nerves and cause pain. However, relief can often be affected by applying pressure for a few seconds on each side of the two muscle tendons at the centre base of the skull.

When the scalp tightens, as a result of tension or anxiety, a person may also experience a thinning or falling out of hair. The tension in the scalp can restrict the blood supply to the hair follicles so that they can often become undernourished. By stimulating the circulation, massage can improve hair growth. It will not make a bald head suddenly sprout hair, but it can improve the condition of the hair. Clients who have had their scalps massaged for ten minutes twice daily, notice a definite improvement in the condition of their hair. The scalp circulation is stimulated and improves, helping to promote texture combined with strength and growth of hair.

Massage of the forehead, or application of pastes such as sandalwood paste, or the application of malai or cream from milk, calms the system and creates good feelings in the brain, making one feel high. Application of sandalwood paste before meditation on the forehead is a common practice in India. It helps one meditate and relax.

The Birthplace and Origins of 'Malish'

There are many schools of thought throughout the East, with each specialising in varying massage themes.

We choose to look at Indian Head Massage, which has a unique place in my life. Known to us as 'Malish', the word is derived from the North of India in 'The Punjab Region', and means simply, *'massage'*.

Malish was a daily activity amongst royalty, and practitioners of Ayurvedic medicine would encourage royals to have treatment for emotional, physical and spiritual growth and stimulation. In ancient times, the study of Ayurveda and spiritual growth was a well respected area and was believed to be one of natures' keys to enlightenment.

The concept of massage began many years ago, when both men and women had long lustrous hair, and massaging the scalp not only helped to promote the strength and vitality of the hair but also encouraged hair growth through stimulation.

The technique of 'Malish' is sometimes part of the hairdressers' service and hair pulling is part of the technique! However, in the West, we might view this differently. Initially, the hair is simply stroked, then a bunch is grasped at the roots and pulled, and although this sounds painful, it does not hurt at all if the hair is grasped in this way. The grasp is released and the fingers are glided up through the hair, and using the hands alternately, this gives a lovely feeling of pulling away all the tightness in the scalp. The ears contain over 110 acupressure points alone, so are one of the most important areas to be massaged. They are also manipulated on a very personal level as an erogenous zone.

Existing ailments are dealt with, but this system too, can be used on a preventative level. Persistent headaches can be successfully treated with acupressure, which aims to unlock the energy in the yang channel of the head. Massage of the jaw line where much tension is stored (which could be caused by clenching of the teeth) may prevent an outburst of negative emotion.

Insomniacs who are given a 10–15 minute massage of the upper back, shoulders and scalp before going to bed should save both parties several hours of interrupted sleep. People who drive for long periods may require

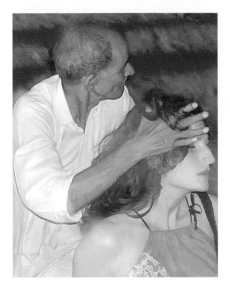

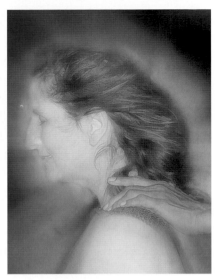

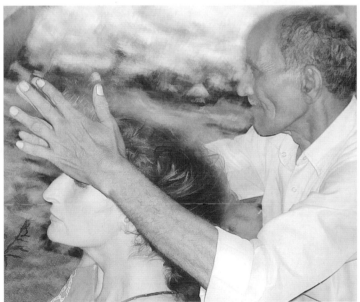

Figure 1: An Indian Head Massage treatment on Chowpatty Beach in Mumbai, India.

more attention to massage of the upper back, whereas those who sit at the desk all day probably will have a more urgent need for specific attention to the neck area.

The Yogis were ancient practitioners of Ayurvedic medicine and they respected the head area as being the most important site for therapeutic massage. Long before the discovery of brain functioning and the progress of neuroscience in the last century, the Yogis believed the head to be the centre of the whole nervous system. They worked their massage around the theory of the brain being the first organ which crystalizes in form in the process of development of the foetus; the head being bigger in size and heaviest in weight (normally it takes three months for a child to balance its head). In childhood, the head has an opening at the top of the cranium where a soft area is present over the section of midbrain. This part is clearly visible, and on closer observation, a recognisable pulsating can be detected. This part is called *'Brahmand'* in Yogic language, and is more commonly known as the *Tenth Gate*.

The body has Ten Gates from which Prana (or energy) leaves:

1.   Anus.
2.   Genitals.
3.   Mouth.
4/5. Two nostrils.
6/7. Two eyes.
8/9. Two ears.
10.   Brahmand (the top of the cranium, about eight finger's width from the eyebrows).

The Brahmand opening is meant to provide energy to the child. Within a period of nine months, this part of the skull becomes stiff and hard like a bone, at which point the opening does not exist. Head massage, very carefully done at this age, is very nourishing. It is only during this period of nine months that through this soft, porous part of the skull, nourishing oils may provide the child with more energy with which to think, learn and remember and have better sight for the rest of his life. After these nine months, not much oil can reach the brain. Head massage done during these nine months energises the cerebrospinal fluid and strengthens the nervous system of the child. This soft spot (Brahmand) is supposed to breathe and absorb Prana, solar radiation and other forms of subtle rays of energy present in the atmosphere. In yoga, this place is supposed to be the seat of consciousness, the seat of self and the abode of self in unconscious-conscious state called *Samadhi*. This portion is directly above the pineal body, the olfactory lobe; the section called the midbrain. This area is in the direct path of the mysterious serpent power (Kundalini) which flows through Shushumna. Application of nourishing oils to this area helps the brain and nervous system.

There are three important spots on the head:

1. The first spot is located at eight finger widths from the eyebrows of the subject, upwards. This is a soft spot at birth; and hardens with the completion of the ninth month. In India (the Northern part), a pad with oil (cotton cloth or cotton ball soaked in oil) is put onto this 'soft' spot, after the birth. This is known as the 'Tenth Gate' mentioned in Yoga scriptures.

2. The second spot is where the 'cowlick' may be found. The hairs at this spot are turning in the form of a whorl; sometimes clockwise, and sometimes anticlockwise. This area is also known as the *'crest'*. Hindus grow hairs in this area; and these hairs are referred to as *'Shika'* (hair grown in a crest/cowlick). This is supposed to be a sign of being Hindu. They twist these hairs and knot them together. This practice is essential for those who practice Pranayam.

3. The third spot is where the neck meets the skull, the place of the brainstem, called the medulla oblongata.

This massage is used on many levels.

Communication

Only a small percentage of communication is carried out verbally; the rest is based on expressions, gestures, mannerisms, actions, and also through touch. Human beings do not touch each other indiscriminately and without motive or purpose. We have developed as a species to be social but also competitive and this has created an interesting concept of communication through touch. When you are next in a public place, take some time to observe the touching which goes on between people. You will quickly see that most developed adults are aware of the concept of each person having something which we tend to term as 'personal space'. We are often very aware of another person's presence behind us, even though we cannot see them and they have not made physical contact with us. We may touch to harm, to reassure, to comfort and to display affection, but no touch is given without an intention to communicate some message to the recipient. No touch is given by mistake. The next time someone touches you, ask yourself what it is that they are communicating to you. Obviously in the ordinary course of communication, you can respond to touch either with a return touch or by other signs and expressions of encouragement (or maybe discouragement).

The head massage is a unique form of touch whereby we are inviting another to give a sustained touch without providing an opportunity to respond in like terms. Unlike the family massage where the treatment is reciprocated between family members, it would be highly irregular for a client to be expected to perform a head massage on the therapist at the end of the therapy. Therefore an imbalance of power exists between the head masseur and the massaged which must be redressed by obtaining and developing trust between the two and learning to communicate on a new level.

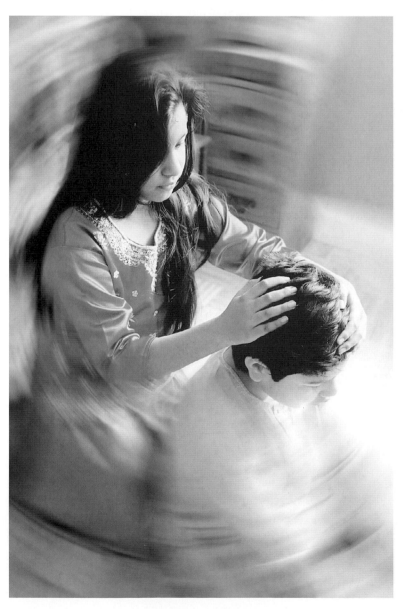

Figure 2: A brother and sister giving and receiving a treatment at a young age.

Many years ago in India when a large percentage of the population were illiterate and only those who came from privileged backgrounds could read and write, most people simply had to rely on the interpretation of truths by those holding the power of literacy. Communication by the spoken word was manipulated by the powerful few to often safeguard their own position. Most people understandably felt a sense of isolation which was relieved by touch. The use of touch signified a certain type of bonding, because we let others into our private space, therefore forming a special communication link. Comfort in touch can be found on many levels:

- A unique bond.
- A personal (spiritual) development within.
- A breakdown of barriers.
- A feeling of focus, clarity and vision.
- An unconditional feeling of rationale.

A bond is formed between daughters and their mothers, fathers and sons and especially grandparents with their grandchildren. Until recently the males of the family groomed each other, as did the females.

Today you can see how the massage is brought down through generations and manipulated accordingly to fit in with the society in which we now live. The males and females also exchange the massage now within professional practice and family.

Things to Consider

- The Indian Head Massage is a tried and tested massage, which has been around for many years, almost since time began, within the Hindu and then the Sikh culture and its traditions.
- Although these methods are very successfully used in the East and now newly applied in the West, there are many things to consider between the East and the West.
- Before applying Indian Head Massage, the main differences between the original Eastern and applied Western approach should be considered.

PMA ('Positive Mental Attitude')

The mental attitude of the East is a very different one to the West with the outlook and disposition being much simpler. The feeling of contentment comes from many simple things, therefore a blessing from faith is a large part of the Eastern philosophy and counting one's blessings means peace is achieved from as little or as much as you have in the material world. The idea of another time after this life allows many who believe, to seek contentment from oneself and those who surround them. As with other cultures and traditions, the focus of achieving one's goals and aspirations comes from the attitude you apply to your life.

The idea of healing and helping others is often appealing to many of us since we too are looking for positive strokes from the work which gives us as therapists a greatly improved positive mental attitude. We can all develop this attitude when we obtain satisfaction that we are using our lives purposefully.

How Can it Help the Therapist?

As many therapists or people involve themselves with helping others will have gathered, there are those amongst us with much more challenging lives than our own. In reality, we come across this every day in some form or another. Our input is seen as a very important one for the client or friend seeking empathy and even solutions.

The short time we spend with others does not give us the right to know what is best for them! However, empathy can be given for whatever discontentment or challenge the client or friend may be suffering. You should always remember that as a therapist or friend, a solution must never be given, since we can never fully understand another person, having not walked in their shoes.

Our very own attitude has an effect on others especially when dealing with those who are discontented. No matter what our own circumstances may be when dealing with others, applying a professional attitude is important. It can be very harmful to our own energy if we allow ourselves to become affected by others.

It is true that we do not always feel on top of the world and even as therapists we need nurturing. A few ideas for keeping a positive mental attitude are:

- A short meditation (*see* page 40) before you start any form of massage or healing process. Taking out time for oneself, a few minutes a day of deep breathing, helping to balance your own energy and bring calmness.

- A gentle exercise regime to release the tension and stress you may be encountering. A simple short walk or yoga can help stretch your muscles and fill yourself with clean air and again bring balance and calm.

- Creating a warm and inviting area to work within. The therapist's place of work is very important for the therapist and for the client. The right environment has to be achieved which is neither too homely nor too clinical. For instance, too much clutter can sometimes be off-putting giving the client a feeling of entrapment, or of unhygienic surroundings. A warm environment can give a sense of security and add comfort, which may help the client to relax. A pleasing surrounding of subtle colours and shades can benefit the therapist, as you are forced to work there. Too many harsh and vibrant colours can cause headaches and nausea for both parties involved. The use of plants is a good way to increase the oxygen levels in the environment during daylight hours but remember to remove them at night. Generally we would like to work in a pleasing atmosphere where we did not feel intimidated by the surroundings and were able to offer our clients somewhere to feel relaxed and at ease.

- Physically imagining all the challenges you have are left outside, until you are ready to face them. There are many faces to life but only one life to face. Although we all have ups and downs in our lives, taking them to work does not help, especially when dealing with sensitive issues! By physically imagining that the whole scenario is outside the door and by creating your own unique space to work within, we can for a short time remove ourselves from the situations which bring us down to earth with a thud. Instead, we can create a space for energising and revitalising both ourselves and our clients.

- Human nature is often very adept at creating scenarios in our minds which can then manifest as physical symptoms and tensions! If we gently begin to change our patterns we can achieve a much more positive mental attitude for ourselves and others around us. If you are feeling tense or troubled, rather than looking upon work as something to be endured, use it to help redirect the mind's energy.

Climate

The weather is a very strong factor in most peoples' lives. All over the world, we are affected by the climate around us. The warm climate, together with the bright sun, channels a sunny disposition and offers a feeling of health and wellbeing. We can also consider some other factors from the East:

- The warm sun feeds the body with Vitamin D, therefore strengthening the bones. This allows more pressure to be applied to the skeletal system for physical labour and intensive work from and on the body.
- The climate also draws out the impurities from the body through perspiration, which in turn cleanses and tones the body.
- Although some food is delicious and very nutritious, the average person in the East would have a small appetite, again reflected by the warmth of the climate.
- The people are left open and approachable which also leads to unity and a good sense of community spirit.

Although we are fortunate to live in a very lush and prosperous country, there are many limitations which are initiated by the climate. The climate would dictate a different approach in the West.

Physical

Due to the limited amount of sunshine that we receive, our physical bodies suffer more as we age. The effect of the cold damp weather can affect our bones, therefore leaving them not as dense, leading to frailty, with ailments such as arthritis and rheumatism. The weather would tend to make us draw in our bodies, changing our posture and sometimes causing us muscular and skeletal problems.

This is one example of why the treatment has to be adapted to fit into the West, to make it effective and beneficial. The pressure applied would also have to be considered at the consultation stage, prior to the treatment itself. If asked what is a gentle, medium or firm pressure, what would you answer?

Although we have our own interpretation of pressure, everybody else's is different. Only individually can we recognise where our pain threshold lies, so the therapist must always be aware of this especially when considering the skeletal and muscular structures of the body. You may have heard the expression, 'no pain, no gain'. This may well be appropriate for work on the limbs and body but is not an approach I would recommend for work on the head region! Working too deep and too quickly means not only hard work for the therapist causing physical exhaustion, but also adverse reactions for the client after the treatment. The theory behind this particular massage is to work slowly with the body's energy and general flow, which should cause no pain!

It is not always easy when dealing with new clients who may be used to the intense pressure given during some body massage techniques and who may suggest lots of pressure initially. However, this task is for the therapist to re-educate the client and to reassure them of the effects of the treatment. As with many complementary/holistic therapies, an immediate impact is not always possible and sometimes a few sessions are required for optimum benefits. However, this therapy does have an amazingly high success rate as an effective treatment.

All the necessary questions at the consultation stage would allow the therapist to carry out a treatment according to the client's needs.

How Does Indian Head Massage Help?

The general state of our PMA ('Positive Mental Attitude') to life and everything concerning it, can be helped along by releasing stress and tension in the back, neck, scalp and face. This is also opening up our clarity and focus of vision.

Combined with a subtle change of our lifestyle, health, personal relationships and work, this makes way for tranquillity, peace and calm, uplifting our level of tolerance for life. The interaction of therapist/client has a comforting effect that can produce a very pleasant and calming feeling.

As with many holistic therapies, we work with a very natural process of eliminating waste from the body, whether it is mental, physical or emotional. A course of treatments is applied accordingly and results can be almost immediate. However, every individual is unique in their own coping strategy and for some, the effects may come more quickly than with others.

Method

There are various methods used in Indian Head Massage. Some of the treatments that I have had whilst travelling in India have been immensely relaxing to the point where I have only wanted to sleep afterwards. Others have been extremely vigorous. It is very much a case of adapting a treatment to each individual's requirements, but also to what would be accepted in the West. The technique that I practice is authentic Indian Traditional Massage, but it is totally acceptable within our more conservative Western standards. The treatment will take about an hour including a full consultation.

Centring

There is an initial very important aspect of becoming centred, focusing totally upon the client and oneself being relaxed. The next essential point is to transfer this calmness to the client by placing your hands firstly upon their shoulders and then by placing your hands on top of the head. This is very reassuring and comforting which makes people feel safe and secure.

The techiques applied on the back, shoulders, neck, scalp, face and ears are a combination of effleurage, petrissage, vibrations, deep kneading and caterpillar movements. Specific techniques may vary, but the overall treatment should follow a pattern so that the massage builds up from the back through the neck and shoulders to the back of head, across the scalp and finally the face.

Initially, the therapist should provide reassurance to the client and engage with their breathing rhythms by placing both hands flat with a firm but light pressure on the client's shoulders. This is generally held for a period of about 30 seconds or until synchronised breathing is established in time with that of the client. The two hands are then placed lightly on top of the client's head to provide a feeling of deep focus and calm. Often clients find this initial contact very uplifting and if it is carried out with care, can induce an early meditative state within the client. If someone is very stressed, the energy coming from the top of the head is tangible and it is important to try to reduce this before starting the treatment, simply by increasing the length of time that your hands remain in this position. When you feel that the time is ready, one hand should be placed on the front of the forehead and the other on the base of the neck for a short while. This can induce a feeling of clarity and focus.

Throughout the treatment, contact with the client is kept either by supporting the head or contact with one hand on the shoulder.

The massage is usually set to music and follows a certain rhythmic flow which helps fine-tune every technique. The treatment allows the client to focus on their innermost thoughts and feelings through the comfort of physical massage techniques, which are a combination of stimuli and relaxation. This allows tension release and depletion of toxins and waste from the muscles.

Some techniques are more invigorating than others and these allow an increase in circulation as well as bringing relief to tired and torque muscles and bones.

Shoulders/Back

The massage treatment starts initially on the shoulders and back with a technique using the whole of the palm to warm the area. Once the area is warmed, a more specific 'caterpillar walk' is introduced using a special thumb technique which travels up the back to the base of the neck. The pressure is gradually increased from light to medium to firm, always depending upon the client's preference of a light or firm touch. A rotation technique is then employed around the shoulder blades, working up towards the clavicle. A friction movement using the fingerpads is then used, stretching the skin to the limits of elasticity. Emphasis is then put on the trapezius area with a technique using the fingers to release the tension that has accumulated there. Finally a pinching/kneading technique is then used over the whole area.

Neck

The next area to be worked upon is the neck. The forehead is supported in the same way as it was initially, and the back of the neck is gently massaged with a special technique using the thumb and fingers. The next technique involves a finger pad friction up either side of the neck. Much attention is then paid to the occipital bone, working on it from two different angles. The Indian 'Malish' Technique is then employed, working along the occipital bone from ear to ear.

Scalp

An extraordinary amount of tension is stored in the scalp which needs to be released. This can be achieved in a variety of ways using both gentle and still motions integrated with more vigorous movements which include shampooing, friction finger pad rub, fingertip circular massage and finally a squeeze and lift technique to complete the area.

Face

The face is then worked on, using minimal touch starting with the temples and then focusing on the acupressure points around the eyebrow bone, the eyes, the nose, the cheek bones and then moving onto the ears, where there are over 110 acupressure points. The cheeks are gently massaged and a sweeping movement is then applied. We then proceed with the laying on of hands closing down the Chakras so as not to introduce any negative energy.

The client is allowed to 'come to' in their own time. They may be so relaxed, that they may not want to go!

Part 2
The Basics of Indian Head Massage

Physical Benefits

- Produces general relaxation within muscles.
- Cells are fully oxygenated; blood circulation is increased and stimulated.
- Release of toxins from tense 'knotted' muscles.
- Neck stiffness can be released by stretching the tissues of the neck and shoulders.
- An increase to the supply of fresh oxygen and glucose to the brain and muscle tissue, providing an increase in the level of overall mental and physical energy.
- Aids in stimulating lymphatic flow and lymphatic drainage.
- The scalp circulation is stimulated and improved, helping to promote texture combined with strength and hair growth.
- Relaxation and harmony bring the body to its own unique homeostasis (balance).
- Massage of the forehead increases eyesight and the power of concentration.
- Massage of the eyebrows relaxes the whole body and is especially beneficial for the eyes and nervous system.
- For young babies and children, head massage can stimulate growth hormones and enzymes necessary for brain development.

As the scalp contains much tension, use of the appropriate massage techniques can relax the area and tone the subcutaneous muscles. This will aid the relief of headaches, eyestrain and anxiety, enabling focus, clarity and concentration.

Psychogenic headaches, which are caused by tension, anxiety, depression and migraines, can often be relieved by this massage, as well as vascular headaches. When the scalp tightens, it often restricts the hair follicles, which then cause them to become undernourished. The stimulation and circulation of the massage helps keep the scalp loose and promotes hair growth. Increased circulation of nutrients to tissues improves the tissue quality and also the condition of hair due to the increased supply to the hair growth region.

Psychological Benefits

- Releases anxiety through the massage of the scalp.
- By creating peace and calm, a sense of focus, clarity and vision similar to a meditation.
- Relief of mental and emotional tiredness, sometimes through a release of extreme emotions, which may be outwardly manifested in either laughter or tears.
- A feeling of rationale and an increased ability and willingness to make decisions.

The Personal Journey

The massage and techniques are only the start of the treatment; once the body begins to become accustomed to its unique balance (homeostasis), then begins a personal journey which takes on the form of meditation.

The benefits are many, but a short list of examples are:

- Focus and clarity of vision.
- Enhanced self-awareness.
- Higher state of consciousness; a state achieved through touch and sound/music therapy.

Every single unique individual has their own personal journey; a balance is obtained through the eyes of the individual, which has no boundaries or time limits.

We find through research and personal observation that once a person engages in a therapy such as Indian Head Massage, it begins to open the mind to possibilities for growth, both mentally and spiritually. The subconscious which we often consider as our intuition is discovered, a direct communication link is opened and a knowledge is developed of what is right for the individual.

There are two certainties in life; from birth we have death and change whether we like it or not. The first is inevitable and we have no control over our mortality. However, we can help instigate changes in life for our physical and psychological improvement. We must first take on this responsibility ourselves so that we may approach change positively and try to welcome new challenges and experiences as part of our personal development.

Through the Indian Head Massage, in addition to the physical feel good factors, we focus on cleansing the mind of irrational and negative thoughts, giving us clarity and vision for our future. This is a process that suits those who like to look that little bit more deeply and develop self-awareness.

Living in the moment and being able to seize the uniqueness of life is a special gift we have, so taking what is ours and making use of it successfully is part of the 'Meaning of Life'. We do not always need to see and feel it to understand.

Stress Management

Stress is an indefinable experience, yet easy to recognise. Stress is often associated with negative images but it is now acknowledged that everyone can benefit from some stress in their day and it is when this level reaches a threshold beyond its benefits that we experience the more obvious symptoms associated with the condition. A racing heart, a small loss of appetite, a sense of alertness and energy are all symptoms of stress; some would suggest that it has similar effects to the feeling of infatuation and therefore could not describe the feeling as in any way unpleasant. It is this level of stress which we are aiming to achieve. That is why we need to be sure that we are trying to manage stress on behalf of the client and not simply eliminate it.

Stress is often experienced internally, so that we are aware the symptoms exist, yet to touch and see them is highly unlikely. Everyday we allow ourselves to have demands put on us which are either positive or negative. However, some are unavoidable, such as work and family. Not everybody has the same stress levels; it is an unspecified response of the body to any demands made on it. Our very own interpretation of the reaction or response we give to any one situation determines how stressed we really are.

Most behavioural psychologists agree that our natural response to a situation can be interpreted as threatening therefore increasing our stress levels on a regular basis with each and every potential interaction with others.

One of the most common stress related complaints is headache. One in three individuals consult their doctor with this symptom every year, and 95% of the population suffers from them at some time. Massaging the scalp, face, neck and shoulders relieves headaches, eyestrain, improves concentration, eliminates muscle tension and helps joint mobility, boosting the immune system and generally creating a feeling of wellbeing. It also eliminates muscle tension and restores joint movement by stretching and mobilising the tissues of the neck and shoulders.

Excessive stress is very harmful, leading to heart, respiratory, digestive and mental disorders. It can also result in muscle tension, allergies and accidents. Occupational stress can also be financially disastrous for organisations whose primary resource is manpower. Continuous stress can lead to more serious and long-term mental illness and more and more companies are looking to provide complementary therapies and counselling services for employees.

Symptoms of Stress

Physical (Effect on the body)	Psychological (Effect on the mind)
Headache or migraine	Tiredness
Indigestion	Anxiety
Raised blood pressure	Anger
Neck or backache	Phobias
Muscle tension	Poor concentration
Addiction to medication or drugs	Depression
Impotence	Low self-esteem
Constipation	Feelings of hopelessness
Irritable bowel syndrome	Irritability/excessive tearfulness

Negative Stress

Some natural expressions of negative stress are:

- Tension.
- Anger.
- Frustration.
- Shouting.
- Tantrums.
- Clenched fists.
- Grief.
- Crying.

However, not all of these traits should be viewed negatively, and the expressions can be determined as either positive or negative responses to stress depending on the perception of the individual producing the reaction.

It is the individual's interpretation of the expression which renders the stress as a negative form. If a person has sufficient self-awareness and control to understand the expression as a form of release, then they will view the stress as being removed from themselves and can understand and enjoy a positive resolution. However, if the person fails to see the reaction as a natural release, then the expression itself can create a further build-up of stress as the initial problem is compounded by a feeling of being unable to cope. A much bigger challenge is set. So we understand that negative stress is an individual's interpretation and can be positive if the recipient understands.

Another concept of turning what is perceived as negative stress into something positive may be to release the tension/stress in a positive manner. Such suggestions are:

- Exercise to release the built-up physical, psychological tension and anger in the body.
- Writing things down so as to look at the scenario objectively before making a rational decision.
- Taking time out for yourself, totally out of your own environment, which can give your own challenges a new more manageable scenario.

Positive Stress

The body's response to stress prepares it for fight or flight, but today's lifestyles do not usually allow us to do either, so the body is left in a tense and alert state. Positive stress prepares you for action and provides motivation to cope with everyday life. Positive stress can be related more to events in our lives that give us a feeling of contentment. For example:

- Annual celebrations.
- A night out with a loved one or friends.
- Retail therapy.
- The start of a new career.
- Starting a family.
- A place to live.

Is it the fact that we are in control of our positive stress that it has a contented feeling? Once again we realise that the individual can cope better being in control of their own stresses and stressors.

What Causes Our Stress?

There are four main factors that contribute to our stresses:

1. Our general lifestyle and status.
2. Our personal relationships, whether with partners, friends and family.
3. Our everyday chores and places of work.
4. Our health issues, strengths and weaknesses.

These affect everybody individually and our place for each factor varies on our age, state of mind, vulnerability and security.

As a very general indication of the above on our growing life, consider what effects you the most and at what time in your life, i.e.:

- Between the teenage years and the early twenties, we may consider 'lifestyle' as a major influence in our lives. Going out, dressing up and enjoying the social aspects of life.
- When we become an adult around our mid-twenties to early thirties, we may consider our 'personal relationships', settling down.
- Once we are settled and maybe start a family, our responsibilities

have an effect on our 'work', which can become a focus for providing for the family.

- As we age, so do the challenges of our physical and psychological wellbeing and our 'health' is now president.

These are very general ways of looking at the major factors in our life. However, we must remember that these are more to do with cultural and social expectations than our biological ones, and we will often come across people whose lives do not fit into our cultural or social view. Care must therefore be taken not to presume or exact our own expectations on our clients.

One of the first laws of nature is 'self-preservation', which is represented by your health. Without this, you would find it very challenging to have the other factors of life. In order to survive a healthy and contented life, the first law of nature should be respected as your foundation to mental, physical and emotional growth.

Aftercare (Short-term) Advice

The design of an individual home care programme is essential for the client to follow, in order to benefit 'holistically' and to accept and welcome the responsibility for self-improvement.

Although very comforting and relaxing, the short-term 'quick fix' provides benefits which are short-lived. As with remedies for the effects of stress, we need to consider and nurture other parts of our lives, looking at the bigger picture to bring about a state of homeostasis or balance. The following advice concerns the client 24 hours during and after the treatment:

- Increase still water as a fluid – at least 2 litres a day. Our stomachs can manage 2.5ls of fluid. A high percentage of our body is made up of water, and therefore exertion on the physical body excretes water and waste. A car does not run unless it has fuel, and therefore our sluggish body depletes unless we top up one of our main fuels.
- Avoid stimulants, for example, tea, coffee, alcohol, cigarettes and drugs. As with many forms of stimulant, it is not always easy to break off a habit of everyday life. However, cutting down can help. One of the benefits of Indian Head Massage is to release waste and toxins out of the body. To make a difference, we must help the body along and not over stimulate.

- Eat a light diet – the muscles in the body are relaxing, including the stomach and to fill it up takes away energy from the body to break down the food. This would also increase tension. Why not try salads, fruit and vegetables? This would also help to rid the body of toxins and waste products. Avoid meats, dairy products and extremely spicy foods.

Exercise to Suit the Client

A gentle form of exercise for the client should be suggested to aid the various systems of the body to work effectively. Nothing too exerting, just a simple approach, e.g. walking, yoga and meditation. The client must remember not to push themselves to the limit.

Breathing Exercises

No one teaches us how to breathe; it is an automatic reflex which occurs without any conscious thought on our part.

As with many skills, one thing we do not learn until we are much older is how to 'breathe' effectively in order to nurture and calm our body and mind.

Deep breathing and centring oneself promotes 'Shanti' (peace and calm). It would be ideal to try this exercise before or during a treatment. The most effective way would be to have some gentle music on in the background and to close your eyes drawing in breath through your nose and releasing it through your mouth. A short meditation is as follows:

Meditation

As a guide you may want to incorporate some gentle relaxing music and be seated upright in a light, uncluttered room.

- No crossed legs or feet.
- Close your eyes.
- Relax, feeling comfortable.
- Deep breaths – in through your nose slowly, out through your mouth slowly.
- Imagine breathing good clear energy – positive thoughts in.
- Breathing out – tired negativity, releasing stresses and tensions.

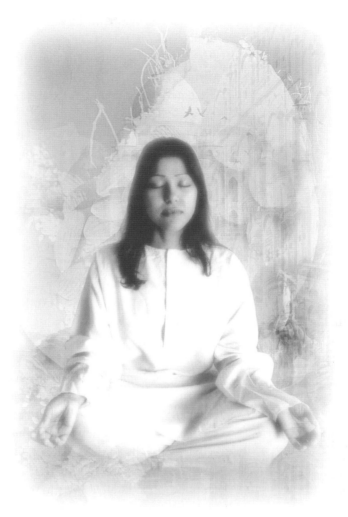

Long-term Advice

As with many therapies, it is important to consider the complete individual, taking account of their overall health, sleeping patterns, eating patterns, careers, activities, age and personal situation. Only then can we devise a programme to suit the individual, which will be manageable for the client to adhere to and work for the client's general health by reducing stress and tension and bringing to balance mind, body and soul.

One aspect of long-term advice would be to encourage a self-nurturing process to comprise the following:

• Regular manageable exercise.
• Applying the correct breathing techniques to create calm and balance.

- To continue with the Indian Head Massage programme for long-term effect.
- Pay particular attention to diet and nutrition, again considering the client's needs.
- Setting aside some time each week for a favourite activity.

As with all advice, the therapist may take the initiative to promote these concepts by applying them to their own lives. The therapist can then more greatly appreciate the problems and pitfalls of their own wisdom!

Adverse Reactions

These are possible after effects of the treatments carried out. They are in no way common to all clients, although they may occur with the individual depending on their constitution and current health. Most feedback is simply positive but adverse reactions do occur and knowledge of these is important for giving client reassurance and explanations. Some of the main examples of adverse reactions are:

- Aching. This may occur during and after the manipulation of the muscles. When tension has been held over a long period of time, the body may hold a different physical posture. Once the massage is carried out and the body relaxes into the natural state, this may cause aching until the muscles become settled. We are also dealing with muscle that may have not had such a manipulated effect on it before.
- Extreme tiredness. Due to the relaxation and change of focus, the body may begin to recognise previous over exertion and stress and the feeling of fatigue is simply the body's attempt at equilibrium. This whole process brings the body to an extreme tiredness which many of us realise when we try to pack too much into the day; when we stop, the body can become very tired almost immediately.
- Heightened emotional state. The nature of this massage is to bring a natural balance to the body, mind and soul. It takes on many forms from releasing stress and tension to bringing a focus, clarity and vision. The fact that we are 'releasing' the body of waste products and toxins means that this also applies to our mental and emotional state, so an extreme emotion such as laughter or tears may take place. This should not be a concern, as any form of 'release' in a controlled way is positive.

It is essential that in good practice, the client is informed first hand of the possible adverse reactions, so the surprise is not felt. Also the therapist may wish to modify the techniques for the next treatment.

In case of adverse reactions, the client must pay particular attention to the aftercare and follow any suggestions made for improvement.

For the Therapist

In order to improve aftercare advice and build a picture of the client's lifestyle on a daily basis, there is certain information required from the client following the treatment:

- How did the client feel after the treatment?
- Had there been anything about the treatment that the client was uncomfortable with?
- What did the client do after the treatment?
- Where and when did the adverse reaction begin?
- How long after the treatment?
- Had the aftercare advice been carried out effectively?

Remember the client does not always realise the reasoning behind questions asked so try to be as specific as possible and consider methods of questioning which you might use in order to get full information from the client – sometimes we have to prompt the client for answers!

Variations on the Indian Head Massage for Clients With Specific Medical Conditions

As with any therapy or treatment, checks should be made on the client's health before engaging in a full treatment. Some medical conditions are often seen as being incompatible with massage. However, variations on the Indian Head Massage can help to enhance a sufferer's wellbeing rather than aggravate any existing condition. The following have been developed:

- High blood pressure. For this, a manipulation of the massage could help high blood pressure by easing and relaxing through deep breathing and using calming strokes in the massage.
- Low blood pressure on the other hand can be stimulated using a more vigorous massage (not too firm).
- Recent whiplash, severe bruising, recent haemorrhage, cuts and

abrasions can be treated using a gentle or modified technique, avoiding certain areas to suit the needs of the client. Naturally some of the areas involved do take time to heal, so particular attention should be applied to this factor or seek medical advice.

- Migraine sufferers are generally aware of their own level of tolerance to pain, and treatment can be beneficial once an agreed technique is planned from the consultation.

Many ailments can be worked upon by the adjustment of the techniques. The massage must be an enjoyable and effective one and not disturbing on any account. Individual clients should be able to confirm their own pain threshold both physically and mentally. Therefore, a full consultation would lead the treatment to be adjusted for the benefit of the client. However, do not always assume that your client will interrupt the treatment massage in order to advise you of an inappropriate level of pressure or touch. During the consultation, therefore, it is wise to encourage them to speak out at any time and reassure them that they should do so even during the massage in order to obtain the full benefit. Only you as a therapist can create the kind of environment where clients feel comfortable in doing this, so bear it in mind when you are carrying out your consultation.

There are many prescribed drugs which affect the body in different ways, sometimes leaving side-effects. Therefore, anything that is new to the therapist should be checked out and medical advice sought if required. Therapists may consider using a medical drug reference list which can give many of the side-effects and contra-indications of commonly prescribed drugs.

Do **NOT** treat the following:

- High temperature/illness/fever.
- Infectious diseases.
- Skin infection, inflammation, etc.
- Localised dilation of blood vessels – aneurysm (commonly the artery in the temple/forehead area within the elderly).
- Intoxication.

Conditions requiring caution (use gentle massage):

- Osteoporosis – not totally contra-indicated, the treatment would need to be adapted using relaxing movements rather than stimulating ones.
- Frailty.
- Chronic fatigue – use only gentle stimulating techniques.
- Avoid spondylitis or spondylosis in the neck. Use of gentle movements only.
- Painful cysts.
- Psoriasis – this condition is not contagious, but caution needs to be taken.

If you do not have the requisite knowledge or skill, do not attempt the treatment! If in doubt, obtain the GP's permission or **DO NOT TREAT!**

The Role of the Complementary Therapist

What is a Therapist?

A question not often asked. However, this is a subject that I feel should be tackled for the benefit of the client as well as the therapist. Although I have fully researched this subject, unless we talk about psychotherapy or counselling, information on the nature of a complementary therapist is limited.

I would like to take an opportunity to reflect on a therapist in the form of an empathetic listener who nurtures the client and who also takes a look at themselves. There are many therapists who come from different backgrounds and have skills that are based on unique training. However, there are some very basic similarities in whatever field we work in. A therapist is a professional who has the requisite skill and knowledge and adequate training in their particular field to carry out a competent and effective treatment.

It is essential that the therapist feels confident in the treatment they are about to apply and follows the instruction of their training. In some professional training, a course of treatments undertaken by the trainee therapist is compulsory prior to qualification. This is not currently necessary to achieve a qualification to practice Indian Head Massage, but it should be seriously considered as part of the training for all students who want to provide a professional treatment.

The therapist has a responsibility towards themselves and their client, delivering information and guidance as requested. It is at this stage that belonging to a membership organisation comes into play. With a reputable organisation, one can follow research and keep up to date with the fast growing industry that is complementary therapy. It also gives you the opportunity to constantly reassess your skills and training, developing your ability to achieve a comprehensive treatment.

A therapist is also looked upon as a professional from whom you would seek individual attention and comfort, as many therapists will realise the client can express the wish to communicate without realising through the divulgence of very personal information. It is not uncommon for initial conversations with clients to reveal extensive personal problems. However, as a professional undertaking a specific physical treatment, we should be careful not to be drawn into this and only work within our professional training and role. Remember we are not there to **DIAGNOSE!** As a suggestion, it would be valuable for the therapist to carry information that may benefit the client such as:

- Other complementary therapies.
- Counsellors or other therapists.
- Citizen Advice Bureaux.
- Professional organisations relating to therapy.

Leaflets and telephone numbers are very useful tools to keep, even a directory giving the client the choice to pick their own suitable way of moving forward.

A professional manner and a comprehensive treatment are all down to the way we are trained and how we use our skills. Therapists must remember to take care of their own physical and mental needs since the work is very physical and mainly conducted over long hours with little fresh air or natural light. Unless therapists take necessary precautions for their own health, they will quickly find their treatments and performance standards falling as concentration levels are lowered and energy is drained from the whole body through the feet.

Emphasis is often placed upon the health and wellbeing of the client. However, this can only be fully achieved after the therapist has ensured that they themselves are physically and mentally in a position to undertake a competent, professional treatment.

The Therapist's Role

We hear the term professional therapist, but what does it mean to you? Think of a time when you may have visited a therapist or even a hairdresser. What were your expectations of the person? Here are a few which are relevant to your practice of Indian Head Massage:

- Carrying out a confident and competent treatment which results in some recognisable benefit.
- Able to assess and understand the needs and to offer advice for individual treatment.
- Able to accurately predict the benefit of the treatment for the client.
- Practice in a clean, pleasant environment, with a degree of privacy.
- Carrying out a treatment which is consistent in quality, making the first of the day as good as the last.
- Comprehensive knowledge of the treatment you are to apply and adequate training. Clients can psychologically feel they are in 'safer hands' if various diplomas and certificates are displayed.

Communication

In the working environment, we must be sensitive to the needs of the client and therefore it is very important that correct methods are used effectively and well, so that communication between the therapist and the client is open and clear.

To be effective, the therapist/client relationship must work on several levels and therefore, all communication must be:

- Concise and accurate, spoken slowly at a reasonable tone (but remember not to patronise your client by treating them like a child with no knowledge or awareness of their body).
- Received and understood by both parties – therapists are not the only ones imparting information and must be aware that the treatment is a two-way process.
- Relevant to the situation.
- Taken by the recipient and acted upon within a reasonable time in the course of ordinary conversation.

Verbal communication with your client is not just about your choice of words but it is also affected by how you deliver your information. Other positive factors that might affect successful communication are body language and facial expressions:

- Facial expressions, such as smiling, concentrating on what is said and keeping direct eye contact. Strangely, you are the last person to have a knowledge of your facial reactions and expressions since the face we see in the mirror is often blank or posed! Ask someone you know well to describe your expressions and see how you might be surprised at what your face has been doing for all these years without you even knowing!
- Gestures, such as slightly shaking the head, confirming and empathising with the client and pointing.
- Sounds of a para linguistic nature and listening, "umm," "I see," "uh huh" are confirmation of listening skills.
- Awareness of individual space, keeping a comfortable distance, sitting not too close, talking with your back to the client.
- Contact of a physical nature, shaking hands, guiding the client to the treatment area.
- Body language, standing straight, slightly leaning forward to listen, hands behind the back and displaying open gestures.

As long as our expressions are not ambiguous, they can be advantageous in the communication process. Just be aware of the expressions you elicit in response.

How Does Being a Therapist Affect You and Your Work?

Are you aware of how your work is affecting you? As a therapist you will be accustomed to listening to people talking about their experiences; not all of them positive. Many therapists can feel overwhelmed and be unaware of the effects such work can have. It is therefore important that stress management is fully understood and mechanisms for coping are developed by individual therapists.

The client plays a very important role in our lives but the first law of nature is self-preservation and without our own health we cannot act effectively for others.

Complementary and beauty therapy are growing industries which allow the client to pamper and treat themselves, but at what cost to your health? Many of us are not sufficiently aware and therefore it is my view that maybe we need to educate ourselves to the dangers of incorrect practice.

My own interpretation of becoming a self-nurturing therapist would be as follows:

- Diet and nutrition – The day is often a long one and a break for lunch is not always possible. At least with a substantial breakfast you will have energy to take you through to the first opportunity for a break. Unexpected events such as late arrivals or some treatments taking longer than others would mean time varying and this is when you begin to play catch up! Throughout the day, drinking water to prevent dehydration and improve our own health. Very often we suggest that our clients eat a sensible diet and avoid many stimulants and heavy meals. Maybe we should take a disciplinary leaf out of our own book!

- Allow enough time between appointments – It is not always possible for the client to be punctual, so allow a little time either side of the appointment. Only fit in as many appointments as is physically possible for the time allocated, making sure the time allocated is not physically impossible!

- Physical, mental and emotional absorption – Many of the clients that visit us have a tale to tell; sometimes it can be quite sad and even remind us of our own personal situation. You may feel at times that the session is stepping into the area of counselling and it is best to develop strategies so this can be avoided. One rule is of course, to never mix business with pleasure! The consequences could be very serious! Next, we listen but do not get drawn into becoming a crutch, which would not only drain you but also take up a lot of your time, which must be considered for others too.

As therapists we are there to aid and help release stress and tension and certainly not to diagnose or advise. We probably would not have the requisite skill or knowledge to do so. This can be dangerous to the client's health and our business/working environment.

Providing relaxation to others is no easy task, and therapists often spend their days on their feet or leaning over relaxed clients. To aid us from physical tiredness and its effects, consider your own body posture. Everyday living would require us to maintain good posture to be effective and not affected. This also holds true in our ability to carry out a treatment. Pay particular attention to your posture whilst carrying out the treatment. If you find the treatment uncomfortable to deliver, then the chances are that the client is picking up the subtle tensions and it is going to have an effect on your body. Why not try a short exercise routine of yoga, meditation or simply taking time out to relax. This can prevent an extreme case of posture-related discomfort and exhaustion.

- Leave it at work? – As therapists, we have joined a work ethic focussed on nurturing our clients, which draws on our empathy and human nature at times. A lot of satisfaction at work is achieved from a client's feedback of a good treatment. It makes the work even more worthwhile and meaningful for us. However, too much contemplation of the day's events can sometimes negatively affect the way we may look at our own personal issues, so try and leave work at work and enjoy your personal life to yourself!

These ideas may not work for everyone, so it is important to develop individual strategies for coping. Remember that, although the emphasis is on being a competent therapist, you are your own foundation and a nurturing process must be followed, otherwise you may crumble!

Although many of us deal with self-preparation on a physical level for the various therapies applied, we really do need to focus on ourselves a little more in order to deliver an effective therapy for the benefit of both client and therapist.

My conclusion is that whilst it is potentially very rewarding, working in the complementary or beauty therapy area has just as many drawbacks as any service industry which relies on human communication. We must try and remember why we chose to be in that particular field in the first place, and ensure that we are gaining all the positive benefits associated with helping others.

The Treatment Area
(Implementing Employment Standards)

The treatment area in which the therapy is carried out can and does have a bearing on the treatment. It is also required by law to conform to certain standards. The points to consider here are based on professional practice either within a therapy clinic or a private home clinic and include health and safety and hygiene requirements.

The General Environment Standard

Is the treatment area clean, tidy and uncluttered? When a client is considering a treatment, it is essential to make the environment comfortable. For this we may take a look at the whole treatment area. Consider warm soft colours on the walls that are pleasing to the eye; nothing that is too harsh or aggressive. Generally, plain pastel shades with a hint of colour are comforting and calming. The therapist is very likely to be working in the clinic themselves and so needs to feel comfortable.

The ventilation of the treatment room is another consideration often overlooked, and although a warm environment is comfortable, we do not wish the clients to fall asleep and miss the treatment altogether. Bear in mind too, that when applying the treatment, the subtle energies used do cause the temperature to rise. Too much of a close environment can bring on tension headaches, so adequate airflow is essential; a good heating source together with an open window is ideal. You will no doubt know of people who are extra sensitive to the heat or the cold and so it is still advised that the client is asked if the temperature is comfortable.

Make sure that there are no potential dangers and obstructions in the therapy room and that all health and safety issues are addressed.

It is advised that music is used to carry out the treatment, so a volume should be chosen which is neither too loud to be an irritant nor too soft that the client is incapable of feeling entirely enveloped in it. No other noise should disturb the treatment and telephones should be disconnected or turned to low volume.

Within your treatment area there are certain tools which you will need:

1. A comfortable chair which is adaptable, depending on the client. Preferably something with a back below the scapula level that has cushioning.
2. A second chair for the therapist opposite the client's chair, for consultation.
3. A trolley close to hand with the following items on:

- Water, for the client and therapist.
- Oils, if used as part of treatment.
- Bowl, for client's jewellery/watch.
- Moisturising cream, for the therapist in case of dry skin (non-perfumed).
- Tissues.
- Consultation sheet/pen.
- Wet wipes.

In addition, a small bin for rubbish close by and a tape/CD player for music whilst carrying out the treatment.

Once contact has been made with the client, it is unwise to leave them unattended, so everything required for a competent treatment should be close to hand.

Some therapists have suggested burning a light oil or incense. However, everybody has their own individual taste and they may not want an oil or incense burning. It could irritate and increase stress through irritation, or even bring on headaches and/or allergies. You must ask the client their preference prior to commencing treatment.

Self-preparation

Having taken so much care to prepare the perfect treatment and environment, this should be continued when considering how the therapist themselves will present to the client.

Professional Uniform

Many organisations and institutions recommend that the therapist wear white clothing. Psychologically, it has been shown that people will respond to advice and commands more readily in situations where the advisor/commander is dressed in a white coat. However, whilst we do seek to gain the respect of our clients, we should not do this by false means. You may therefore think that 'whites' are not appropriate in delivering a service which seeks to empower the client and encourage them to take more responsibility for their own wellbeing. As with other organisations, promoting professionalism and hygiene is key for any therapy, but the colour of the uniform has to be given consideration. White in my opinion relates to allopathic treatments delivered by doctors and dentists and can unleash fear and tension by its relation to an unpleasant incident the client may have experienced. The colour black can also effect the treatment, relating it to a negative event. With this in mind, I suggest a light pastel colour, which will not intimidate or have a negative reaction from the client. We still keep our professional image, yet promote a more humanistic approach to the therapy; after all, it is holistic and nurturing. Many people's healing, as doctors will tell you, is psychologically based and is heavily reliant on the belief of the patient in the doctor and/or therapist. Imagine yourself arriving for an Indian Head Massage. What would you like to see the therapist wearing to instil confidence and belief in their healing powers?

Appearance

The main concept to understand here is that of cleanliness. We begin to consider our appearance as a whole, with the hair being neat and tidy, tied up and out of the face. All nails should be short, with no nail varnish, and the hands should be clean and warm at all times. Because some of the techniques used come into close proximity on and to the face, you must respect the client's senses. For example, if you apply creams to your hands, make sure they are not perfumed, as this could put off the client or irritate the client's sense of smell, as would smoke on the hands and any form of perfume on the skin. Make sure your breath is also clean and not off putting, as once again you are working in close proximity to the face.

This may seem rather obvious, but because the client is sitting comfortably with their eyes shut, the perception of the other senses is heightened and enhanced; such as smell, touch and taste. When working with subtle energies, all the above should be given special consideration prior to treatment.

Do not wear any jewellery, as this can interfere with application of the therapy and scratch the surface of the skin and any cuts or abrasions on the skin must be covered by clean plasters. These are both hygiene standards.

The Consultation

As all forms of complementary therapy grow and become ever more popular, a professional and standardised approach is needed in Indian Head Massage to monitor the treatment outcomes and therefore offer clients a treatment that best meets their needs. When carrying out a consultation, remember that all the information given by the client must be recorded concisely and accurately. All information given to the client must be clear and effective – steer clear of pseudo medical jargon as much as possible and find other ways to obtain your client's confidence in your ability to help them.

In applying a treatment of Indian Head Massage, we need to gather as much information as possible before we begin the massage. The initial consultation could take anything up to half an hour and includes consideration of medical history, both past and present. But the consultation for the therapist can start even earlier, at first contact whether it is a phone call or a meeting to book an appointment in the diary.

Initial Contact and Information

Head massage can be beneficial at any time, except for the time immediately following food and other conditions under which massage is prohibited. It is especially good in the morning before bathing and if necessary, in the evening after having finished work for the day. Obviously as a therapist you will not want to be taking too many 6am appointments, and so you will have to establish which time of day is most appropriate for you to work and for your client to obtain the full benefit from the treatment. However, it is helpful if you advise them in advance of the booking, not to eat for up to two hours before the treatment, if possible.

At first contact, there are many observations to be made. Although your client could be a little nervous or anxious, there are other considerations. For this, let's start with the following:

Body Posture

- What is the posture of the client like? Is it upright or slant over?
- Is it open or closed, confident, or vulnerable and insecure?
- Would you consider it to be positive or negative towards you?

The fact that a client could be suffering from backache, stress and tension or some injury, may well be reflected in the posture. It would then affect the way the client walks. An observant therapist will therefore already have an idea of which area to focus the treatment around and where to avoid and adjust the pressure as appropriate. Any obvious back problem needs to be addressed when seating the client. At this point we can suggest something suitably comforting, which would still allow access to treat the upper back.

Whilst we consider the posture of the client, we should also pay attention to their body language. Negative and uneasy body language could present as any one of the following:

- Lack of direct eye contact.
- Folded arms and a tense posture.
- Apprehension.
- Frowning.
- Shaking the head.
- Foot tapping or drumming fingers.
- Impatience through para linguistic sounds such as 'tut tut' or sighing.

Although the above can be disturbing for the therapist, we must react positively (as suggested in 'The Therapist's Role') so as to ease our client into relaxation. We soon find that our positive manner and body language has an effect on the client and therefore creates a bond, making it less challenging for future treatments.

The Medical Consultation

Once we have introduced ourselves and what the treatment is all about, we are then in a position to carry out the medical consultation, which is normally written on a pre-designed sheet or card. This must include all the relevant medical history and data required by the therapist before the treatment can be carried out.

The medical consultation sheet can be as comprehensive as you feel is necessary, considering the whole treatment time allowed. Some required points to include are as follows:

- Personal details – Name, address, telephone number, date of birth and occupation.
- Doctor's details – Name, address, telephone number and whether the doctor's permission is necessary before treatment is carried out, where relevant, for clients with specific medical conditions.
- Various ailments and specific medical conditions – The following list should be checked with the client: diabetes, epilepsy, asthma, respiratory problems, allergies, dysfunction of the nervous system, skin diseases/disorders, heart problems, blood pressure (high/low), kidney/liver problems, thrombosis/embolism, high fever/infection, oedema (i.e. swelling), severe bruising, recent haemorrhage, cuts and abrasions, recent fracture/sprain, recent operations, metal/pins/plates, spinal disorders (e.g. slipped disc), arthritic pains, muscular aches and pains, headaches, nausea, current medication, possibility of pregnancy, phase in the menstrual cycle (and whether regular).
- To what degree do you indulge in the following? – Smoke, drink alcohol and exercise.
- Indemnity clause – It is important that the client has given you all the information that is necessary for the treatment to be carried out effectively. Therefore, the responsibility is on the client and an indemnity clause ensures that all is understood and accepted. This also promotes a professional contract which can be perceived as a legal document.

It is essential that the medical consultation is completed by the therapist and not the client. All the various ailments and specific medical conditions should be explained, so that the client understands them. Medical terminology can confuse, so the therapist should also be aware of the ailment or medical condition they are talking about and be aware of its effects.

Other information can be written on the medical questionnaire such as special diet or food intolerance and lifestyle factors which make up an everyday routine. The whole consultation is a record of the client, and can be used by the therapist to adapt treatments if necessary and keep an account of the client's personal development for future consultation.

The consultation should continue after the treatment, in order to keep proper records of the feelings during and after the treatment. It is also a point where the relevant aftercare advice can be suggested and a leaflet may be presented to the client with information regarding the advice and possible adverse reactions for the next twenty-four hours.

Remember that the consultant sheet is a confidential document and therefore must be locked away in a safe place and only consulted upon with colleagues after permission by the client.

The Treatment

Once the initial introductions have been made, personal and environmental standards observed, and the medical consultation been established, we can then begin the practical treatment. You should be aware of all the relevant information required to carry out the treatment, including any adaptations needed. The treatment can be broken down into:

1. Assessment of the client for Indian Head Massage – From our consultation, we must now have information regarding general health, specific medical conditions and general lifestyle of the client, including hobbies, diet and occupation. At this stage, we also know why the client is having the treatment.

    The information provides the therapist with an outline of the treatment, and any areas to concentrate on are now established.

2. Application of Indian Head Massage – It is essential that the client is aware of the areas you are going to massage, as they may feel uncomfortable with certain parts of the treatment plan. Some clients do not like their ears being touched, whilst others may have severe pain in an area or even a psychological problem with physical contact. Therefore an outline of the massage is necessary, so that the client is not made to feel uncomfortable.

    Before the massage, think about the techniques you are about to use and their effects. Is it going to be beneficial to the client and is there any need for you to adapt the treatment, techniques or the way you deliver the movement?

Whilst you are applying the massage, try not to become automated, but remember to concentrate on each movement and the corresponding desired effects.

What is the client expecting as an outcome of the treatment you have applied? At the initial treatment it is normal to have some benefit, but this is because there is a detraction of focus caused by the client being unable to anticipate the next movement. Subsequent treatments should allow the client to relax further without this distraction and obtain the full benefit.

The length of treatment should be limited so as not to overstimulate and/or inflame any problematic area. However, a deeper treatment can be applied with the consent of the client if required.

3.   Evaluating the Indian Head Massage Treatment – After completion of the massage, the therapist can evaluate the treatment for the benefit of their own professional development and for future treatments carried out on the particular client.

Was the client happy with the treatment and did it fulfil the objectives as an effective treatment? For future reference, would you adapt the treatment applied for a more effective outcome? Would the client return to you for another treatment? All these questions are beneficial for your development and must be considered when applying the next treatment.

Other considerations may come from observing the client's body language. Remember that it is essential at this stage to give positive aftercare advice and explain any adverse reactions that may occur.

A full evaluation may be better obtained by calling the client after a few days and discussing the effect of the treatment with them at that stage.

As with any other complementary therapy, no two treatments are alike and each client has individual expectations and individual outcomes. The therapist must deliver an effective treatment, benefitting each client individually, and so must be constantly adapting and concentrating on the client's requirements.

Case Studies

As part of the learning process for students, the practical and theoretical sides of Indian Head Massage are explored in case study work. This is then used as a measure for the assessment criteria. These case studies can be used as part of any course assessment in the study of Indian Head Massage and most courses incorporate up to three different studies before professional level qualification is obtained. To achieve the most competent treatment for the client, we focus on case studies to help us understand how the therapy works before we deliver it within industry.

How Does it Help You as Students?

By continuous repetitive practise of the practical treatment, we are able to deliver the massage techniques with confidence and can concentrate on the different pressures required. Case studies allow you to work on a variety of individuals, applying different approaches and pressures according to the individual's needs and characteristics.

The case studies emphasise the fact that the massage has to be specifically adapted on each occasion; each massage should be as unique as the person receiving the treatment.

There are several points which need to be covered in order to meet the assessment criteria:

1.   A profile – This is a basic description of the client and includes age range which can be broken down into: young (up to and including 40), mid-range (up to and including 60), mature (over 60).

      You need to be aware of the flexibility of these boundaries – we all know people who act much younger or older than their chronological age.

      The profile should also include a brief description of what the person does for a living, with particular reference to the stress and tensions involved. Once again, you should try to avoid stereotyping occupations with stress levels and remember that everyone has their own level. Some people may find light housework stressful yet take a demanding intellectual career within their stride!

You may also want to look at a person's hobbies and interests which may give you an idea of how the person may release some of their stresses and tensions and how active they are in their daily life.

The profile may also contain any ongoing medical problems which affect the person on a day to day basis.

2.   Observations – Observations recorded in the case study are useful in allowing tutors and assessors to build a picture of the client from your case study. They give character to your profile and allow the client to exist as a more three-dimensional person. They can also act as a prompt to some physical condition which may be recorded on the consultation sheet, allowing you to adapt the treatment as necessary and help to consider the development of the client from initial contact to improvements occurring after several treatments.

The more you develop use of perceptive observation, the more you will be able to practice as a holistic therapist taking your client in totality rather than the sum of unrelated parts.

3.   Recording Treatments – Each session is written up in detail to provide evidence that you have considered health and safety issues, professional appearance and comfort of the treatment area. Obviously in practice you would not be expected to record all of these features, but simply the ones relating specifically to the individual and the treatment, so we will start with these.

4.   The Specific Treatment – Before any treatment is begun, the client needs to be assessed, taking into account any health problems or other contra-indications specific to that client. The case studies should reflect that this has been covered even where no problems arise. At this stage, the outline of the treatment can be planned and discussed with the client before delivery.

It is important to record how the treatment was carried out, if there were any specific adaptations to the treatment, and the expected results. You should record which areas you massaged, and which movements you used in the treatment. Remember that you will also have to perform the treatment in a commercially acceptable time if you are to offer the treatment professionally, and so the length of time taken also needs to be recorded here.

Although you may already have observed some apprehension in a client's body language at the beginning of a treatment, you may like to ask the client how they are feeling and what they expect from the treatment. This will serve as a useful record for future treatments. You should also record any observations of the client during the treatment which may affect any future sessions. For example, it is not uncommon for clients to experience nausea during massage.

Many clients will comment on their immediate reaction to the treatment, often very positively, and this should be recorded as far as possible. This is where we can consider how far our objectives have been achieved and how effective the treatment was for the client. This is part of the evaluation and allows consideration for the provision of aftercare.

5. Summary – This comprises detailed evaluation of the treatments carried out in the case study, considering the results which have been obtained after the total number of treatments. This is where we investigate the reactions of the initial treatment against the reactions of the final treatment, and identify the development and progress for this particular case study.

    This is essentially a record of your opinion as to how the treatment has benefitted the client based upon your own understanding, perception and observation of the client prior to and after treatment.

    The summary should also serve to increase your confidence as a practitioner in seeing how beneficial Indian Head Massage can be and allow you to advise future clients based on your own experience of delivering treatments.

6. Self-evaluation – Rarely do we ever act perfectly, and the student of Indian Head Massage is no exception. The purpose of self-evaluation is not to be critical for its own sake but as a personal tool for the practitioner in continuing development and improvement of the art. These methods allow you to see how your application, confidence and intuition develop from the initial treatment; by allowing this critique of oneself, you can build your own confidence and deliver more competent and effective treatments in the future.

7.   Testimonials – A testimonial is a handwritten letter from your case study client to you and your course tutor which confirms that they have received treatment from you and explains any benefits which they may have noticed as a result. It can also simply be a letter stating how much they enjoyed the treatment even though they could not identify any benefits. The testimonial should be left until after all the treatments for the individual case study have been completed.

As an alternative, you may want to consider allowing your case study client to dictate this information to you after the final session and have them sign and date the letter at the end.

Case study clients are generally family and friends who are supporting you during your studies, and it is important that they understand that confidentiality will be maintained, since you will be recording personal data about their health and other matters. In practice, you will need to identify your clients by their name and also have a record of their address. For the purposes of your studies, this is not necessary, and it will be sufficient to give your case study clients false names and addresses to observe that confidentiality.

Example Case Study

A consultation has taken place with client X and a consultation card completed, which records the following points for consideration:

Medical conditions	**Medication**
Sinus problems	Contraceptive pill
Headaches	Fluoxetine
Low blood pressure	(seratonin reuptake inhibitor)
Arthritic pain	
Nausea	

Profile

X is a single professional young woman in a high powered job. X works long hours and travels up and down the country for her work, often staying away from home. She therefore encounters a lot of tension through driving, long hours and the nature of her work, which is mainly dealing with demanding clients in difficulties. Her work does not allow any time for hobbies and interests except for some walking which she has been unable to do due to the recent closure of local footpaths.

To release stresses and tensions, she has in the past found going to the gym beneficial but recently the membership has lapsed because she feels that she cannot justify the fees with her attendance being so poor.

There has been nothing severe in terms of her medical history. However, recently she has been taking medication for increasing seratonin levels, which have the effect of relieving the major symptoms of depression. Her sleep patterns have been disrupted for the past year and the medication has not relieved this problem.

X tries to adhere to a regime of five pieces of fruit and vegetables each day and finds this quite easy until she has to start travelling around, when she eats a lot of convenience snack food at service stations and cafes. She drinks about five cups of tea per day and has a couple of glasses of wine in the evening. Her water intake is low.

Observations

X's appearance is that of a confident, well-groomed, articulate young lady who takes pride in her appearance and holds her posture upright. There are signs of direct eye contact and much humour in her tone. However, there is a slight apprehension about the treatment and this is noted through the body language, which is slightly restless. The communication is clear and X understands the full procedure of the treatment and what it involves.

Although she is taking medication for depression, she appears to be quite cheerful but obviously does not want to talk about the condition and is somewhat reluctant to mention the medication at all in the beginning.

Treatment Write-up

Preparation

Preparation for health and safety issues will depend on whether the client is to be treated in their own home or in a clinic. Obviously more consideration will need to be given to these matters where you are going into a client's home, as it is unlikely that they will have set up any area of their house with the same considerations in mind. In this case, X was treated in her own home.

Prior to the treatment, X was asked to provide a room or area that was well-ventilated, with adequate heating and which was also private and away from disturbances. For health, safety and hygiene requirements, the room, which X had chosen, was checked for any potential dangers such as trailing wires or obstructions. A large space was cleared around the chair in order to carry out the treatment comfortably. The chair itself was checked for height, comfort and back level (just below the shoulder blades) on the client.

The items required to carry out the treatment were placed on a small table within easy reach and they comprised of: two glasses of water, wet wipes, tissues, bowls for jewellery and rubbish, pen and consultation sheet, unperfumed moisturising cream for the hands. In the corner of the room, a CD player was set up to play gentle and relaxing music at a low volume.

Consideration was given to my own appearance, and I ensured that my hair was tied back, my nails were short, my hands were warm and smoothed with moisturiser and my breath was fresh. I had not worn any aftershave prior to the treatment. I was dressed in a cream coloured polo shirt and navy blue trousers in order to look smart and professional without appearing too clinical.

The Specific Treatment

X was assessed as having low blood pressure and she also mentioned that she is hypersensitive to the cold, so the temperature of the room was increased to a higher than normal level in order to compensate for this, and to ensure that she would remain comfortable throughout the treatment. It was also suggested that she put on some socks or slippers to maintain the temperature of her feet.

The full treatment was discussed and it was indicated to X exactly which body areas would be touched during the treatment and explained the different pressures and techniques to be used. Since she had no bruising or other skin contra-indications, the full treatment could be carried out without any specific adaptations. After looking at the consultation sheet, I advised X that I would pay particular attention to the face massage because of her sinus problems and I would also pay particular attention to the back, neck and around the occipital area to release stresses and tensions. All the pressures would be light yet stimulating movements, because of the low blood pressure.

Client's Feelings Prior to the Treatment

This was discussed with X who confirmed that she was looking forward to the treatment and expected to feel more relaxed afterwards. The body language did appear a little apprehensive, but this may have been due to the fact that this was her first Indian Head Massage.

The massage was performed in a commercially acceptable time of thirty minutes and the three types of pressure were used. During the treatment, X seemed to relax very quickly and soon her body language suggested that she was in deep relaxation. All the techniques were used and there were no problems with any of these. However, I did note much tension around the upper back and neck area. The scalp itself seemed torque around the top, which is normal. However, after applying different techniques, it seemed less tight.

After the treatment, I asked X to come round in her own time and offered her a glass of water. After a couple of minutes I began to question her on feelings experienced during the treatment.

Client's Feelings During the Treatment

X said that she felt the massage to be very soothing and relaxing particularly around the back of her head. She was surprised at the lightness of the touch and had, at the time, wished that it was firmer in places not realising the effectiveness of the treatment.

Client's Feelings After the Treatment

X was surprised, given the light touch, at how different she felt when the treatment was finished. She said that when she opened her eyes again it was like waking up from an anaesthetic or a very deep sleep. X said that once this feeling had gone, she was left feeling lighter and with sharper vision with a heightened sense of colour.

At this stage I carried out the aftercare advice and explained to X about the adverse reactions that could occur. I was mindful of the fact that she had previously disclosed her proneness to headaches and advised her that she may well experience these symptoms following treatment due to release of waste toxins from the body, and that drinking plenty of water would help eliminate these more quickly.

Three treatments were carried out each with different outcomes and a final summary recorded the investigation.

Summary

Initially, X was slightly apprehensive and did not quite know what to expect, even though everything was explained. For the final treatment, X knew exactly what to expect and seemed much more relaxed going into the treatment and was able to reach an even deeper understanding of the therapy through the level of relaxation she achieved. This was very obvious from the discussions we had after the treatment regarding the different colours and feelings X had experienced. In my opinion, X has had to make some changes to her lifestyle in order to lessen the stresses and tensions which had built up and which were unconsciously part of her life. During the course of the treatment, X has been able to focus on more fundamental aspects of her own self and has begun to adapt her life accordingly, through the development of new directions and goals.

Self-evaluation

On the first treatment with X, I felt a little bit nervous as it was the first time I had performed the treatment outside class and did not have the tutor support on hand. I had also not met X before and so was not as relaxed as I had been in class when using the techniques on other students. I felt that our initial consultation was rather stilted, with me feeling as if I was just going through a list of quite intrusive questions. I think that in future, a different technique would have worked better where I could talk to a first client more informally in order to get much of this information rather than looking like a market researcher on the high street.

Our second and third meetings were much better and I think that this was because of the familiarity and the relationship which had developed. I felt more confident on these occasions due to developing more competence of the techniques through practise. I have learnt that much of my nervousness as a student practitioner on case studies came from not only my own lack of experience and confidence but also from clients' expectations that I will know everything about the Indian Head Massage treatment. In this case on the second meeting, X became more interested in the therapy and began asking me a lot of questions that I could not answer. My impulse was to make something up but resisted and told her instead that I wasn't one hundred per cent sure, and that I would check on the information for the next meeting. I thought that she would be disappointed but she didn't appear to mind and I had all the information ready for her on the final visit.

Testimonial

To whom it may concern

I have been asked to write this testimonial on behalf of the therapist to confirm in writing that I have had three Indian Head Massages from him/her on the following dates:

March 5th 2001
March 15th 2001
March 23rd 2001

I have enjoyed the treatments and have been impressed at how effective they have been in relieving stress and encouraging relaxation.

In particular, I have noticed that I am sleeping much better now, and am following the aftercare advice leaflet which was given to me to help detoxify.

Case Study X
March 23rd 2001

(This case study may help give you an idea as to how the written assignments should be completed. It is not given as a comprehensive case study due to client confidentiality, which has meant that some details have been left out. It is to be taken as an example only).

Part 3
Anatomy and Physiology

General Massage Considerations

Muscle tension indicates that the muscle is working even when the person is relaxing. It can develop as a result of particular activities, protective reactions after trauma that have become habitual, attitudes to life, or via a slow and often unconscious accumulation in response to the demands of life.

If muscles are constantly tight, blood circulation is restricted and they do not function as well as when they are relaxed. They are working and consuming energy for no good effect, which is tiring. It is harder to be active because the muscles have so little potential for movement. Initially, tight muscles are sore, but over time, they usually become less sensitive. General massage techniques will work well in these conditions, supplemented by deeper work if you are trained to apply it.

Tension often accumulates in lines in the long muscles of the limbs and the wide muscles of the trunk, which can be addressed most effectively by using techniques that knead the muscle and stretch it in various ways, and also pressure strokes. In shorter muscles, such as the network of muscles alongside the spine, where there are commonly knots of tension, pressure strokes may be most useful as it is harder to move the muscles around.

What Does Massage do for Muscles?

Even a friendly touch on the skin may be calming for some people, encouraging them to relax and this may encourage some muscle relaxation

As we age, we tend to accumulate tensions in our muscles and they, along with many other body tissues, tend to dry out. Massage is one of the ways of halting and reversing this sequence. Massage can help muscles to soften generally and can be applied to specific adhesions to reduce or release them. Softening will help the muscle's own blood flow. Kneading and sliding pressure strokes can actively pump blood, lymph and other fluids through the muscle.

When a muscle becomes tight, the fascia around it will also shorten and stiffen. These adhesions can be addressed by myofascial and deep tissue techniques.

However, if you think that muscle tightness is protecting a weakness or an injury, be cautious in your approach, or refer the client to a person trained in dealing with such injuries.

Some bodywork systems use the reciprocal inhibition of antagonistic muscles to promote release in tight muscles and/or rebalance between them. If a muscle is tense, tightening the antagonistic muscle will encourage it to let go. While a chronically tight muscle may need relaxation, the antagonist may need to be stimulated.

A number of approaches also make use of other reflexes. For example, in Proprioceptive Neuromuscular Facilitation (PNF) a muscle is taken to its comfortable limit and then contracted against a resistance that prevents movement; it can then often be stretched further by the practitioner.

Massage, either through techniques applied directly to the muscles or via passive movements that stretch the muscles, increases the potential for flexibility.

Initially a massage practitioner wants to be able to work effectively on muscles, but after a time, many practitioners want to search out and address the deeper causes and habits that contribute to muscular tension. A person's tensions and postural habits develop gradually from his activities, injuries and accidents, and are also shaped by the person's attitude to life and his feelings and beliefs. Massage, in addition to the physical effects described above, can help to increase the client's awareness of his tensions, allowing him to consider ways of reducing these tensions and changing physical and attitudinal habits that encourage the accumulation of tension.

Muscles and Massage

As you gain experience in identifying muscles on people of different builds, you will find that you can also begin to identify tension in the muscles. Over time this will allow you to assess the level of tension in an individual's muscles, comparing it to your developing experience of the common distribution of tension throughout the body for someone of similar age and build.

When you have explored the bodies of a range of people, you will start to sense the effect of repetitive or constant job or leisure activities. Massaging people of varied ages will help you develop a feeling for the slow accumulation of tension over time that comes from postural habits, sedentary lifestyles, and/or responses to injuries. You'll begin to gain a sense of how each person uses their body.

This developing feeling can extend beyond merely sensing how your client's physical activities and postural habits affect his or her body. You may also start to gain an appreciation of how their attitude to life affects their body, i.e. how they live in their body. A worrier, for example, may develop a fixed frown or be constantly fidgeting and be unable to relax. Be wary, of course, of glibly reading meaning into every tension you encounter in your client's body. And make sure that you listen to their thoughts and feelings about their tensions, rather than making rigid assumptions.

Therefore, as you massage, it is worth keeping in mind that massage may do more than just encourage the recipient to release some of the tension they have developed through activities and physical habits. As they let go of some physical tension, they may also let go a little of some of the attitudes that contribute to the tensions, even if it is only for the duration of the massage session. In the case of the worrier, for example, their forehead may smooth out and they may feel more relaxed and less concerned than usual. This is one of the reasons why people can feel a little dazed after a massage; they are not quite 'themselves', i.e. the way that they are used to being. Attitudinal habits are referred to in the section that describes the muscles of the face, as this is the area of the body where they are most obvious and are often the major cause of tension.

Where there are references to massage strokes or to exercises given to clients, these are general suggestions about what would be appropriate for the average person. It is assumed that readers will adapt these to suit the recipients, being guided by their build, injuries, sensitivities, muscle tone and their responses.

Physiology of Massage

Many claims are made regarding the benefits of massage, and the positive effects that it can have on the body, mind and emotions. How accurate or well-founded are these claims? There are two aspects that need consideration. One is that we need to be specific about what we mean by 'massage'. Sports massage, 'holistic' massage, Swedish massage, lymphatic drainage and myofascial release all involve manual manipulation of the soft tissues, but use different techniques, with varying degrees of pressure, to achieve different results. Even a stroke with a generally accepted meaning such as effleurage can be performed in diverse ways; consider effleuraging a back very quickly, with minimal pressure, and then imagine doing the same stroke using your full body weight, slowly. Even though your hands are moving identically both times, the affect on the underlying tissues, and the feel of the strokes to the receiver, are very different.

Also, to what extent can claims about the effect of massage be backed up by research findings? When we notice the skin on someone's shoulder reddening during massage, we assume that this is due to localised vasodilation, bringing more blood to the surface of the skin as capillaries dilate. However, it would be inaccurate to claim from this observation that this proves that massage improves circulation. All we can say is that, for that person, on that day, the techniques we were using caused vasodilation in the skin on the shoulders. Generalised statements like 'massage improves circulation' are meaningless until we have evidence-based research. This might include flow in arteries or veins or capillaries that are observed consistently when measured before and after a massage – stipulating duration, type and amount of pressure. And then we might want to know how long the change in circulation lasts and whether it is temporary or permanent.

This section attempts to address these problems by categorising massage strokes in order to provide a framework to relate these to the possible effects of each category of stroke on the physiology of the body. It then looks at the possible effect of massage on the different systems of the body. The categories are not definitive and other practitioners of massage might use the terminology differently.

There is a growing body of research that does validate some of the claims that have been made concerning the affects of massage. All massage therapists know that people sometimes fall asleep during a treatment, and assume therefore that massage has a relaxing effect. From this we could also assume that massage stimulates the parasympathetic nervous system. We could even try to work out the likely pathways between touch and the relaxation response. Now, with evidence that massage reduces levels of noradrenalin and cortisol, two hormones associated with stress, there is some scientific back up for the claim (Field, et al., 1999).

Some of the claims made in this section have scientific validation and some are theoretical; given our knowledge of the body as it is at the moment, this is what may be happening.

Although at this time we cannot say for certain how a particular touch effects the body in terms of the exact input / response pathways, we can speculate. The effects of massage are mediated via the communication systems. Put very simply, when the therapist touches the receiver's body, the touch is registered by sensory receptors in the skin, joints or muscles and messages are relayed to the spinal cord and up to the brain where they are processed. As a result, messages flow down the spinal cord and via motor nerves to the skeletal muscles. At the same time, neurotransmitters are released at the synapses, the neurochemical balance in the brain also responds to the incoming information, and the homeostatic balance of the body is subtly altered. Memories of previous experiences of touch are stimulated in the cortex of the brain and this information added to the neurochemical response. The balance of the autonomic nervous system is affected.

Some of these input-response routes have been carefully mapped. We understand how a reflex arc works, for example the path taken when the patellar tendon is tapped. There are hypothesis regarding other effects of touch, for example the 'pain gate theory'. Other effects, particularly those involving the messenger molecules in the body, we can only guess at this stage.

Categories of Massage Strokes

Classical Swedish massage defines five types of stroke: effleurage, petrissage, friction, vibration and tapotement (percussion). Additional techniques now widely in use are holding, feathering, compression, trigger points and passive movements. Strokes are classified here according to the level of tissue activated as well as the broad technique involved.

1. Holds – One or both hands in contact with the body, no or minimal movement, and minimal pressure.
2. Stroking, feathering, light effleurage, light vibration – Strokes that engage the skin and subcutaneous tissue (superficial fascia, capillaries and lymphatic vessels).
3. Deep effleurage, petrissage, kneading, compression (palming), trigger points – Strokes that engage the muscles, using a rhythmical compression and release of the tissues.
4. Skin rolling, connective tissue massage, friction – Techniques that address the connective tissues.
5. Percussion: hacking, cupping, tapping, pummelling – Techniques that use repeated rhythmical light striking, and affect the skin, connective tissue and muscles.
6. Passive movements: stretches, shaking, rocking, joint mobilisation – Techniques hat involve movement of muscles in relation to bones or joints, or joints in relation to the torso. The structures engaged are the muscles and joints.

Massage strokes and sensory receptors affected:

1. Holds – Hair end organs in skin on limbs, free nerve endings and Merkel's discs to light touch. Thermoreceptors to heat.
2. Stroking, light effleurage, feathering, light vibration – Hair end organs in skin on limbs, Meissner's corpuscles in non-hairy skin and free nerve endings.
3. Petrissage, kneading, deep effleurage – Stretch receptors in muscles, Golgi tendon organs in tendons. Ruffini's endings to deep pressure.
4. Skin rolling, connective tissue massage, friction.
5. Percussion: hacking, cupping, tapping, pummelling – Paccini's corpuscles, and Meissner's corpuscles to light percussion.
6. Passive movements: stretches, shaking, rocking, joint mobilisation – Ruffini's endings and Paccini's corpuscles in joint capsules, Golgi tendon organs in tendons, stretch receptors in muscles.

Pathways between sensory receptors and the brain:

1. Sensory receptors to spinal cord then to one of two ascending sensory pathways.
2. Vibration, light pressure and touch, and the kinesthetic sensations from stretching and movement of body parts are transmitted through the rapid transmission pathway.
3. Information about the body at rest, tickles, itches, sexual sensations, crude touch and pressure, temperature and pain are transmitted through the other pathway, arriving at the brain more slowly.

In the brain:

1. All information is transmitted through the brainstem to the thalamus for sorting and then sent to other parts of the brain.
2. The somatosensory cortex in the parietal lobes registers that part of the body is being stimulated.
3. The association, or memory cortex and existing neural connections relating to touch are stimulated. Existing patterns of responding to touch are activated.
4. The release of neurotransmitters affects the balance of the autonomic nervous system. The HPA axis reduces output of stress hormones.
5. If negative thoughts are acting as an internal stressor, a shift to more positive thinking also reduces sympathetic nervous system activity.

Pathways from the brain to the body:

1. Information is transmitted back to the body through the descending motor pathways in the spinal cord.
2. Motor neurons that have been firing persistently, and maintaining skeletal muscle fibres in a state of contraction, are inhibited and the degree of contraction reduced.
3. The parasympathetic nervous system is activated by the vagus nerve and heart. Respiratory, digestive, urinary and sexual functioning is affected.
4. Reduction of ACTH from the pituitary reduces adrenalin output from adrenals.

Figure 3: The bones of the head.

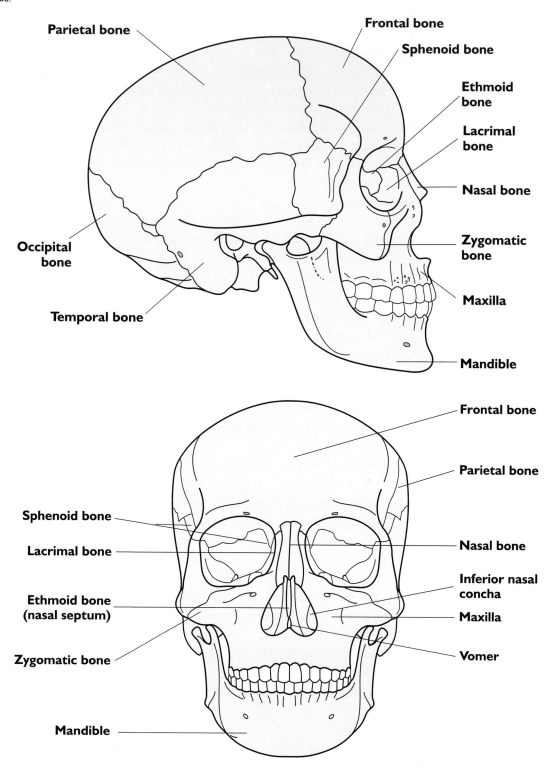

Bones of the Head, Neck and Shoulders

The head is made up of eight cranial bones, fourteen facial bones, the hyoid bone in the throat and three tiny bones called ossicles in each ear, which are part of the hearing mechanism. Each ear and most of the external parts of the nose are made of cartilage.

The cranial bones form a solid container, the brain 'box' that surrounds and protects the brain. The inner surface is lined by membranes, the meninges, that in turn contain a fluid. Together, these cushion the brain from jarring against the bony cranium in the course of ordinary daily activities. There are many small holes through the bones for the passage of nerves that connect mainly to the muscles and sensory organs of the head.

At birth, these bones have soft areas of membrane called 'fontanelles' between them to allow the baby's head to adapt to the birth canal. As the child grows, all the bones of the skull gradually grow together along 'sewing' lines called 'sutures', except at the connection between the upper and lower jaw. The bones of the top of the skull are relatively smooth and evenly curved. At the front, the frontal bone makes up the forehead and the upper part of the eye socket. The cranial bones below it spread back under the brain, forming part of the nasal cavity and connecting to many of the facial bones.

The back surface of the skull, from about halfway down, is formed by the occiput (occipital bone) which also forms the posterior part of the underside of the skull. This under-shelf extends quite some way under the skull, providing a large area for the attachment of the many layers of muscles in the neck that hold the head upright and move it around.

Towards the front of this under-shelf is the large hole called the foramen magnum through which the nerves of the brain stem exit from the cranium to form the spinal cord. In four legged animals, this hole is much higher on the back of the skull. Because we humans stand upright, it is directly under the skull.

In front of the foramen magnum, there are two small bumps called condyles on either side, via which the occiput sits on the first vertebra. The head can rock on these to give a small nodding movement – nodding 'yes'.

Between the frontal bone and the occiput, two parietal bones join at the top and extend about halfway down each side. Below them at each side of the head, a temporal bone extends from the temples back to the occiput, and some distance under the head. It contains the ear hole and also forms the back part of the cheekbone. Just behind the ear, there is a lump of bone under the skull called the mastoid process, which serves as an attachment place for muscles. 'Process' is a general name for a bony projection and this one looks a little like a breast, so it is called mastoid, meaning 'breast-shaped'.

The front of the skull is formed by the facial bones. They are all strongly interlinked with each other, apart from the lower jaw, forming the bony surface underlying the face, the front of the cheek bone, the bony parts of the nose, the upper palate of the mouth, and the upper jaw – the maxilla.
Many of these bones contain sinus cavities that make the bones lighter. These are hollow spaces, some of which are lined with mucus producing membranes. Those close to the nasal cavity are connected to it and contribute to a person's vocal quality. 'Sinusitis' is the condition in which they become inflamed, usually due to upper respiratory tract infections.
The lower jaw, the mandible, is the largest and strongest of the facial bones. It is the only bone of the head with any significant mobility, apart from the hyoid. There are two large muscles that move it for the important activity, in terms of survival, of chewing. It forms a joint with the temporal bone – the temporomandibular joint (TMJ). When the jaw is held tight, TMJ problems can develop, including grinding the teeth, aching jaw and headaches.

The hyoid is a small, horseshoe shaped 'floating' bone. It is not attached to any other bones, but is held in place by small muscles that form the base of the mouth and the front of the neck. These muscles move the hyoid when a person swallows. It also serves as a base for some of the muscles of the tongue. Because it is commonly removed with the muscles in dissection, it is often missing from display skeletons, and also quite often from illustrations of the full skeleton.

Muscles of the Head, Neck and Shoulders

The muscles of the head that can easily be massaged are thin, flat muscles, either wide sheets of muscle or short straps. Apart from the jaw muscles, most have only small attachments to bones and pull instead on other soft tissues.

The scalp muscle covers the top of the head, spanning from the forehead to the occiput.

Facial expressions come primarily from the actions of the small straps of muscle that pull and stretch the three oval muscles of the face, one around each eye and one around the mouth. The muscle around each eye only has two associated muscles, but there are many going to the mouth to help shape vocal sounds and expressions. In addition, there are small muscles that knit the eyebrows and wrinkle the nose.

There are two large chewing muscles on the outside of the mouth that are important in massage. The base of the mouth is also formed by muscles, which can be massaged just behind the mandible.

Although the face is a small area of the body, there are a large number of motor and sensory nerves to this area, controlling and monitoring the range of expression that we use for communication. Thus, a significant part of our brain is concerned with this area. We often hold much tension here, and a good face and scalp massage can have a beneficial releasing effect that is disproportionate to the area covered.

Because of the importance of the face in communication, tensions here will often be related to responses to events or attitudes to life, especially those around the mouth and jaw and to a lesser extent the eyes.

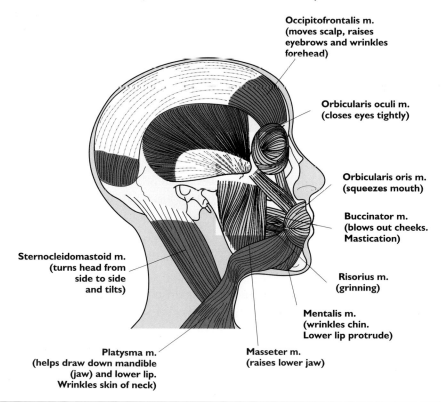

Figure 4: The muscles of the head.

Occipitofrontalis m.
(moves scalp, raises eyebrows and wrinkles forehead)

Orbicularis oculi m.
(closes eyes tightly)

Orbicularis oris m.
(squeezes mouth)

Buccinator m.
(blows out cheeks. Mastication)

Risorius m.
(grinning)

Sternocleidomastoid m.
(turns head from side to side and tilts)

Mentalis m.
(wrinkles chin. Lower lip protrude)

Platysma m.
(helps draw down mandible (jaw) and lower lip. Wrinkles skin of neck)

Masseter m.
(raises lower jaw)

Scalp

Occipitofrontalis: The muscle of the top of the scalp (also known as the epicranius) consists of three parts:

1. A short muscle at the back attached to the occipital bone (occipitalis);
2. The short frontalis muscle at the front attached to the muscles above the eyes, and;
3. A long aponeurosis joining them (the galea aponeurotica).

Its potential movements are small, acting via these short muscles fibres at each end either to pull the scalp forward or backward, or to raise the eyebrows. When you massage over the top of the scalp, you can usually get some movement in this muscle, although in some people it seems to be held fast. At the front, it overlaps with the muscles at the top of the nose, and those just above the eyes. This is one of the few muscles that straddle the centreline of the body.

Facial Expression

The nasal muscles: Corrugator (corrugator supercilii) and procerus are two small muscles that join to the occipitofrontalis just above the bridge of the nose. They draw the eyebrows down and together, in expressions of frowning or puzzlement. Nasalis covers the lower half of each side of the nose, widening or narrowing the openings of the nostrils.

Sensitively performed, massage across the forehead and around the bridge of the nose can give the recipient a feeling of opening out in this area and, for a while, can relieve the pressure of a frown or sinus congestion.

Around the eyes: Each orbicularis oculi muscle ('orb-shaped of the eye') is attached to the bones around the eye socket in a few small places and has just two short 'straps' of muscle that move it. Much of its movement comes from its own sphincter-like activity – squeezing in on itself in parts, e.g. in winking, closing the eyelid, or squeezing the tear ducts.

These muscles should not be worked on directly, but they relax when the surrounding muscles are softened through massage.

The mouth: In contrast to the eye muscles, the orbicularis oris ('orb-shaped of the mouth') is not attached at all to bones. It is held in place, stretched and moved (in vocalising, sucking or for expression) by a number of strap muscles that attach at their outer ends to the bones of the skull. Some called levators lift the upper lip or the corner of the mouth, e.g. in smiling. Some called depressors pull down on the lips or the corners, e.g. in an expression of sadness, and orbicularis oris itself can tighten or purse the lips, allowing us the range of expressions of which we are capable.

Singing teachers and theatre voice coaches often comment on the mouth tension that they encounter in their students, and it seems common for many of us to hold our lips stiffly much of the time. Massage can again play a role here in releasing, at least for a short time, habitual expressions and tensions.

Platysma, which covers the lower face muscles and then continues down the front of the neck, is described more fully in the section on the neck.
The cheek: Buccinator is a thin, square muscle that stretches between the mandible, the maxilla and the orbicularis oris to form the inner lining of the cheeks. It moves the food between the teeth in chewing. It also compresses the cheeks when they have been stretched, so it is important in blowing; its name comes from the Latin word for a trumpeter/bugler.

Chewing Muscles (Muscles of Mastication)

There are two muscles on the inside of the mouth at the back (the pterygoids) that masseurs ordinarily do not work on, but the two larger ones on the outside are important for massage practitioners.

Masseter is a relatively short but strong muscle running between the corner of the mandible (jawbone) and the cheekbone (the zygomatic arch of the temporal and zygomatic bones). It is easy to palpate at the back of the cheeks when it is contracted.

Temporalis runs from the top of the mandible, behind the cheekbone, to the side of the head, where it attaches to the side of the skull above and round the ear, behind the edge of the temple. You can often usefully work with pressure on this muscle, but you also need to exercise care, as it can be quite sensitive at times of great stress, when the accumulated tension can lead to headaches spreading from the temples and around the side of the head.

These muscles, which are so essential to masticating food and are also involved in speech and singing, need to be strong for the amount of work they do. They can also become jaw-clenching muscles when chronically tight. We tense them when we put on a 'social face', e.g. a polite smile when we don't feel like it, push ourselves hard (when we 'grit our teeth') or hold back from expressing feelings ('bite back our words'). Many people hold considerable tension in the jaw muscles, which shows itself as unconscious grinding of the teeth at night, waking with an aching jaw, or headaches.

Muscles of the Neck

The main muscles of the front, sides and back of the neck control the position and movements of the neck and the head.

In the lower part of the front, the sternocleidomastoid muscles cover the infrahyoids. At the side of the neck are the scalenes that act as side 'guy-ropes', stabilising the side to side balance the neck.

At the back, trapezius, which forms the outer layer, and its associated underlying muscle, levator scapulae, raise the shoulders, and are involved with other muscles in moving the scapula.

Under trapezius, the splenii muscles in turn cover the top section of the deep postural muscles of the back, the erector spinae, and the small para-vertebrals that form the network of fine-tuning muscles between adjacent vertebrae.

Just under the base of the skull are the very small sub-occipital muscles that control the small nodding and turning movements of the head.

All of these muscles, by their actions of balancing and stabilising the neck, respond to movements from within the head, such as chewing or will stiffen with lack of neck or head movement. Suboccipital tension can often be related to eye tension, and can be a step in the build up of headaches; headaches can also be related to jaw tension. Tension in the neck, especially in the lower cervical region, can be a consequence of tension in the back and shoulders. And of course tension in all these areas can be due to injuries and/or part of postural habits.

Front of the Neck

The infrahyoids form the front of the neck below the hyoid bone. The sternocleidomastoid (SCM) covers the lower parts of the infrahyoids.

The main part of the SCM extends between the top of the sternum and the mastoid process of the occiput, just behind the ears. A short fork at the lower end goes to the clavicle – the 'cleido' part – not as easily visible when the muscle is relaxed, but able to be felt, and usually seen, in action. This gives the sternocleidomastoid a secondary leverage point for the movements of the head that it controls in coordination with other neck muscles – especially the scalenes, splenii, levator scapulae and the upper trapezius.

Depending on the actions of these other muscles, one SCM can act to turn the head to the side – the right SCM turning the head to the left and vice versa; it is easy to see on the exposed side of the neck in this action. The SCM also helps in bending the neck strongly to one side.

If both sides are working, it is a major flexor of the neck, tilting the head towards the chest, but it can also play a part in extension (tilting the head backwards). It is sometimes called upon to play a part in forceful inspiration, raising the sternum and clavicle at the front to increase the ribcage area.

When massaging this muscle, do strokes which stretch it lengthways or that lift it away from the underlying tissues. Avoid applying pressure that could affect the structures that it covers, particularly the windpipe, which lies between the 'V' shape formed by the two SCM's, and the carotid artery that carries the main blood supply to the head.

Platysma covers the SCM and the infrahyoids. It is a thin sheet of muscle that stretches from the muscles on the lower side of the lip to those covering the upper chest. It can pull the outer corner of the mouth down in an expression of aversion or wrinkle the skin of the neck. It is the same muscle that a horse will twitch to flick flies off its neck.

Side of the Neck

The scalenes are three muscles (anterior, medius and posterior), deep in each side of the neck. They run from the transverse processes of most of the cervical vertebrae (C2–C7) to the first and second ribs. The lower parts can be palpated at the side of the neck, in the angle formed between the back of the sternocleidomastoid and the front of trapezius.

These are the side 'guy-ropes' for the neck, holding the neck and head upright or working more strongly on one side to tilt the neck and head to that side. They can also be involved in forceful inhalation by lifting the ribs.

They are tight in most people, especially those who spend a lot of time at a computer, or working at a bench.

Back of the Neck

The outer layer of the back of the neck is formed by the upper part of the two trapezius muscles, which are involved in stabilising the neck or conversely in raising the shoulders, either on one side only or both together.

The name refers to the collective shape of the two muscles, which together form a trapezoid – a kite shape. The trapezius muscles are attached along the centreline of the neck and the trunk – to the occiput, the nuchal ligament in the cervical area and all the thoracic vertebrae to T12. They stretch to the shoulder girdle, attaching to the outer third of the clavicle and the whole top edge of the spine of the scapula.

The upper section runs between the outer part of the shoulder girdle and the cervical spine. The structure of the rest of the muscle and its role in movements of the scapula is covered in detail in the next section on the muscles of the shoulder and the arm.

If the shoulders are held still by other muscles, one side of the upper trapezius can either act with the same side SCM to turn the head to the opposite side, or with the scalenes to side bend the neck (pulling the head down on this same side). The head and neck can be bent backwards by the simultaneous action of the upper part of both trapezius muscles.

Figure 5: The lymph nodes of the head.

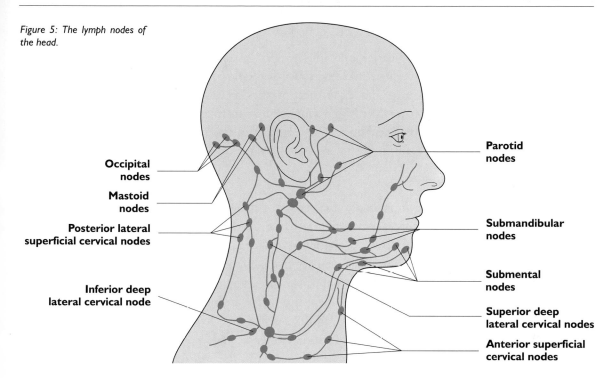

Occipital nodes

Mastoid nodes

Posterior lateral superficial cervical nodes

Inferior deep lateral cervical node

Parotid nodes

Submandibular nodes

Submental nodes

Superior deep lateral cervical nodes

Anterior superficial cervical nodes

The Immune System and Adaptive Immunity

The organs and tissues of the immune system, which provides specific immune responses, are the red bone marrow, the thymus gland, the spleen and the lymphatic system.

Red bone marrow is the site of manufacture of all blood cells. In the infant, red marrow is found in all bones and in the adult, mainly in the ribs, sternum, vertebrae and pelvis. As well as erythrocytes (red cells) and platelets, there are six different kinds of white blood cells. Those involved in acquired immunity are called lymphocytes. Some remain in the bone marrow to mature (B cells) while others travel to the thymus gland for programming (T cells). Most of this activity occurs during infancy, when the thymus is proportionally very large; after puberty it stops growing although it still produces T cells.

As part of the circulatory system, the lymphatic ducts of the lymphatic system filter intercellular fluid back to the heart from the tissues through the lymphatic ducts. On route, the lymph passes through several lymph nodes. The ducts begin as tiny, open-ended tubes, picking up fluid and wastes that haven't returned to the capillaries from the tissue spaces. Flow of lymph, like venous blood, depends on suction and muscle pumping.

The capillaries join into lymph vessels, which then feed into the main lymph trunks that lead towards the heart. Lymph in three trunks from the right arm and right side of the head and chest drains into the right lymphatic duct. Four lymph trunks from the rest of the body feed into the large throacic duct. The lymph fluid from these two ducts drains into the two subclavian veins, just below the clavicles, to rejoin the main circulation.

The lymph nodes are masses of lymphatic tissue inside a fibrous capsule. The spaces between the tissue are full of white blood cells that ingest waste, bacteria and foreign material. When there is an infection to deal with, white blood cell activity increases, the nodes swell up and may feel sore. When this happens, we complain of 'swollen glands'. (From a structural point of view the nodes are not glands at all, since they don't produce hormones, sweat, sebum or saliva but act as filtering stations). The nodes mostly occur in clusters in the neck, armpit and groin, and deep in the abdomen.

The spleen consists of masses of lymphatic tissue, but unlike the lymph nodes that filter lymph, the spleen filters venous blood. The white blood cells in the spleen ingest not only waste, bacteria and foreign matter but also damaged or old red cells and platelets.

Nearly all organs and tissues (the central nervous system, bone marrow and cartilage are exceptions) contain lymphatic tissue. The sites of entry into the body are guarded by lymphatic patches of tissue. The tonsils at the back of the throat and the adenoids under the tongue are made of lymphatic tissue that protects the upper respiratory tract. In the intestines, sites of lymphatic tissue are called Peyer's patches. The specific immune response, involving the cells and tissues of the immune system, is activated when the inflammatory response fails to contain infection, or a disease-producing substance gets past other innate defences, and enters the circulation or lymphatic tissue.

All foreign matter, bacteria, viruses, toxins, and pollutants have molecules called antigens attached on the outside of the cell membrane. If the body has encountered a particular antigen previously, a memory of that antigen is activated in the lymphocytes and an attack mounted following one of these two routes:

1. Humoral immunity is where B cell lymphocytes produce antibodies, which are chemicals that circulate in the blood, recognise antigens and trigger a variety of destructive responses. This includes clumping of cells to hinder movement within the body, or direct invasion and cell death.

2. Cell mediated immunity is where T cell lymphocytes summon other white cells to infected areas and the antigens are destroyed by phagocytosis.

Immunisation is a way of creating artificial memory in the immune system. There are two kinds; in active immunisation, a very small harmless amount of an organism is injected into the body, and the immune system develops antibodies to it. When the organism is encountered again, these antibodies recognise it and attack. In passive immunisation, blood from a person or animal who has recently had the disease is treated so that the antibodies are separated out, and these are then injected into the body. Passive immunisation is used when someone has risked exposure to infections such as tetanus or rabies.

Skin, Touch and Massage

Our skin is the boundary between what is inside us, our blood and guts, and what is outside. We become very aware of this fact when the boundary is breached, and a bit of inside spills over into outside. Skin is also a psychic boundary, the point where all that I think of as 'me' stops and all that I think of as 'not me' begins. Once upon a time as very small babies, none of us were aware of that separation; we all had to learn it gradually.

Skin, together with eyes, ears, nose and tongue, provides us with information about the outside world. With over half a million sensory nerve receptors embedded in its surface, skin is our largest sense organ, weighing approximately 3kg and covering an area of 2m². As part of the nervous system, the skin is constantly sending information to the brain. Right now, your brain is registering the contact of clothes on different parts of your body, the pressure on the skin of your legs and buttocks (if you are reading this sitting down) and the temperature of the air around you. This information is filtered through your memory; your perception of all this might be different from another persons'. There is evidence that early experiences of touch determine how we understand touch when we grow up. There are implications here for the massage therapist. And, since it is the surface that we contact first, before muscle, fascia or bone, a knowledge of the structure, function and conditions that affect the skin is essential to the massage practitioner.

The skin consists of three layers of tissue, within which are found nerves, capillaries, hairs and exocrine glands. The whole organ, skin and appendages, is known as the integumentary system.

Structure of the Skin

The skin consists of three layers of tissue; the most superficial is epithelial tissue, and underlying that are two layers of connective tissue. The epithelial layer is called the epidermis, in contact with the dermis, there are sheets of epithelial cells, plentifully nourished by blood and continuously replacing themselves. The next layer is the dermis, connective tissue with loosely arranged strands of collagen and elastin fibres, which give the skin its elasticity and mobility. The last layer connecting skin to fascia is the hypodermis, also called the subcutaneous layer or adipose layer, a layer of adipose tissue which is connective tissue with fat stores.

Figure 6: The structure of the skin.

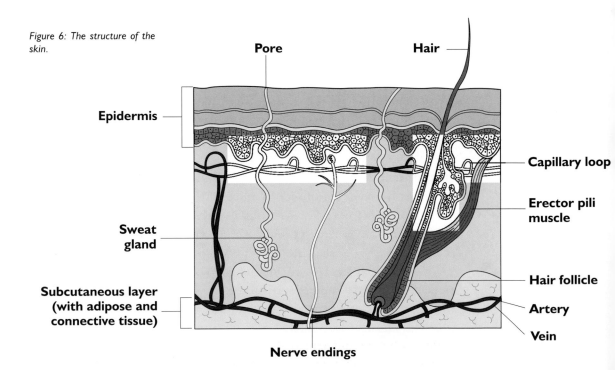

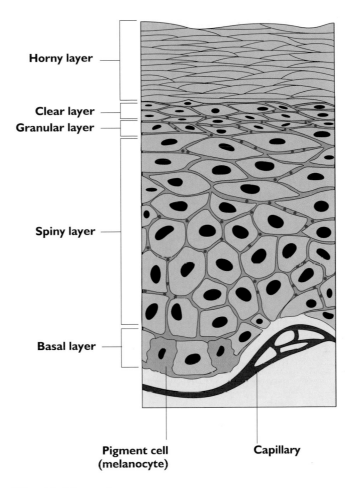

Horny layer

Clear layer

Granular layer

Spiny layer

Basal layer

Pigment cell
(melanocyte)

Capillary

The Epidermis

When looked at under a microscope, it is easy to identify two aspects of
the epidermis. One is that it is composed of sheets of cells, one on top of
the other, and that the structure of the cells alter as they get further away
from the dermis. The other is that the base layer of the epidermis is not
flat, but has a corrugated appearance, with lots of bumps protruding into
the dermis. These bumps are called papillae, and their function is to
increase the surface area of the deepest layer, called the germinative layer.
This is where new epithelial cells are constantly being formed by division
of existing cells. The capillaries in the skin only reach to the germinative
layer, so the nutrients required for cell function are no longer available as
the cells divide and get pushed towards the surface. The pigment melanin,
which gives the skin its colour and protection from the ultraviolet rays of
the sun, is produced here. Exposure to the sun increases both the amount
and the colour of melanin.

In the next identifiable layer, the granular layer, the cells are beginning to flatten, and deposits of a chemical called keratin, which is waterproof, are being formed. By the time the cells have passed through the clear layer, and then the outer horny or cornified layer, they are quite dead, flat and full of keratin. These outermost cells are constantly being rubbed away; we replace the whole of our outer epidermis every four weeks.

The cornified layer has important protective functions; the dead cells form an impenetrable barrier to bacteria and viruses, unless cut. This is one of the body's routine defence mechanisms against disease. Areas of the body that are exposed to continuous friction are protected from damage through the development of a thicker cornified layer in the epidermis. The soles of the feet are the obvious example; callouses on the hands of workers using certain tools are another. The ends of our fingers and toes are protected by nails, which are horny plates of cornified epithelium growing out of the epidermis.

The Dermis

Interspersed in the ground substance of the dermis are the organs and tissues that impart to the skin its multifunctional aspect; the blood vessels and lymphatic ducts, the nerves, the hairs, and two sorts of exocrine glands. The blood vessels consist of networks of fine capillaries, which fill each papillae, bringing blood to the surface of the skin, and to the germinative layer of the epithelium. Each hair follicle and gland also has its own capillary network. These capillaries are connected to arterioles and venules deeper in the tissues of the body.

Hair grows most plentifully where it is needed to trap sweat or protect the skin; on the head, eyebrows, armpit and groin. Each hair grows in its own sheath, or follicle, attached to which is a tiny muscle, the erector pili muscle. These are involuntary muscles, which contract in cold temperatures, causing the hairs to stand up away from the surface of the skin. This traps a layer of air, which has an insulating effect. These muscles also contract as part of the fight or flight response; in mammals, fur standing on end gives them a larger and more threatening appearance.

Sebaceous glands, a type of exocrine gland, secrete an oil called sebum, that keeps the hair and skin moist and pliable. Sebaceous glands mainly open into the hair follicles. Overproduction of sebum at puberty is one of the causes of blackheads and acne.

The other kinds of exocrine glands in the dermis and adipose layer are the sweat glands. These are found all over the body except in the lips and nails, but are larger and more numerous in the palms, soles, forehead, groin and armpit. They are coiled glands with a duct passing up to open on the surface of the epidermis. They secrete sweat, which is a combination of water, salt and traces of other wastes, to cool the body by evaporation.

Effects of Massage on the Different Systems of the Body

Musculoskeletal

Massage that kneads and squeezes the muscles relieves stiffness, spasm, and tightness in the area massaged. The movements are detected by Golgi tendon apparatus and stretch receptors in muscle and tendons.

Fluid circulation is improved, wastes including lactic acid, the cause of muscle stiffness, are removed and oxygen and nutrients delivered to the muscles more effectively, and muscle functioning is improved. Light massage that interrupts the pain cycle may result in a decrease in muscular spasm. Percussive strokes cause an increase in muscle spindle activity in the immediate area, causing minute contractions in the muscle fibres and improved muscle tone.

Joint manipulations may facilitate production of synovial fluid in an under-used joint. Local massage around a fracture seems to facilitate formation of scar tissue and healing in bone.

Connective Tissue

Deep massage may flatten out adipose tissue in the skin temporarily. Restrictions and thickening in fascia, tendons and ligaments may be relieved. There are specific techniques for reducing adhesions from scar tissue in fascia.

Nervous/Endocrine

Depending on the techniques used, the autonomic nervous system is stimulated or soothed. Massage that relaxes stimulates parasympathetic activity, resulting in a decrease in anxiety, perceived pain and improved sleep. Pain is affected both by release of endorphins, neurochemicals that act as natural painkillers, and by the decrease in sympathetic nervous

Figure 7: The superficial main nerves of the head and neck.

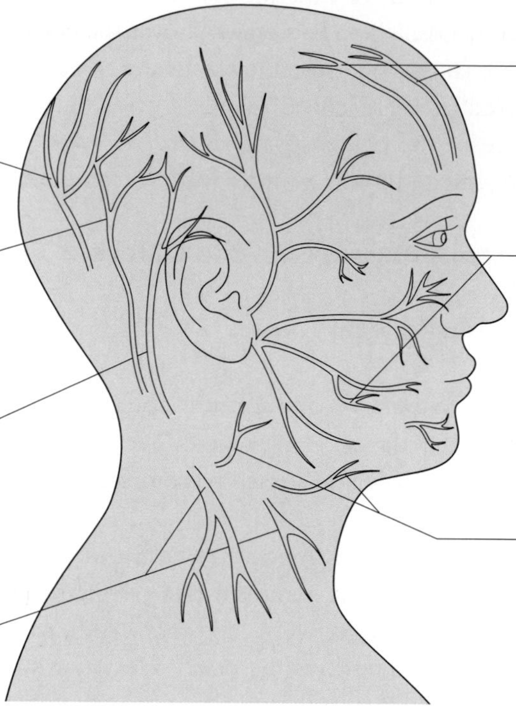

Supraorbital nerve

Greater occipital nerve

Lesser occipital nerve

Facial nerves

Great auricular nerve

Transverse cervical nerve

Supraclavicular nerve

system activity, and by massage interferes with the nociceptive pain pathways in the spinal cord. Trigger point techniques relieve localised pain by improving fluid circulation in that area.

Cardiovascular

Draining and deep effleurage assists venous flow locally by mechanically pushing blood through the veins. The superficial circulation is increased by techniques that cause localised vasodilation of the capillaries. Both of these facilitate delivery of oxygen and nutrients and removal of waste.

Dilation of the capillaries temporarily decreases blood pressure. As sympathetic nervous system activity decreases, heartrate drops. There is some evidence that massage facilitates production of white blood cells and therefore ability to fight infection, the theory being that the body perceives massage as a micro-trauma and releases white cells to deal with it!

Lymphatic / Immune

Massage mechanically stimulates lymph flow in ducts and improves circulation of lymph through nodes. There is some evidence that massage facilitates production of white blood cells and therefore the ability to fight infection. Relaxing massage decreases sympathetic nervous system activity, and as levels of cortisol drop, allergic and inflammatory responses are restored.

Skin

The superficial circulation is increased by techniques that cause localised vasodilation of the capillaries. Sebaceous glands are stimulated and sebum improves texture and tone. The rise in superficial skin temperature results in improved evaporation of sweat from the surface, and removal of wastes. Certain massage techniques can reduce the formation of keloid and scarring in soft tissue.

Respiratory

Relaxing massage decreases sympathetic nervous system activity and respiratory rate slows. Massage of the intercostal muscles and diaphragm attachments can improve ribcage mobility and the mechanics of breathing. Compression, vibration or percussive techniques on the ribcage can loosen phlegm.

Digestion

Relaxing massage decreases sympathetic nervous system activity and improves digestive functioning. Clockwise massage on the abdomen may alleviate constipation mechanically and may stimulate peristalsis.

Urinary

Relaxing massage decreases sympathetic nervous system activity and improves urine output.

Gentle Massage

There are certain client groups for whom 'gentle massage' is recommended; with the very elderly, with people who are frail after long illness, or women in the late stages of pregnancy. Gentle massage may be suggested locally, even when the rest of the body can be treated normally; over thin skin or over areas of oedema. What does it mean? It is obvious that the holding and light contact strokes (light vibration, stroking, light effleurage) could be considered gentle massage, but all the other techniques could also be performed in a gentle way. Percussion with the fingertips and minimal pressure, as used on the face, for example is gentle massage. Kneading performed slowly and lightly could be considered gentle massage. The main points to remember is that the massage should not require a big response from the body, and should aim to activate the parasympathetic nervous system. The attitude and intention of the practitioner to perform a careful and caring massage is possibly as important as the choice of techniques and the degree of pressure employed.

Structure and Function of the Respiratory System

Air enters the body through two nostrils of the nose, and/or the mouth, and passes immediately into the nasal cavity, which opens out behind the nose, above the roof of the mouth. The epithelial tissue lining this part of the respiratory tract is covered with fine hairs, or cilia, and also contains secretory cells, which produce mucus. The mucus traps unwanted material like dust, or pollen, and the waving motion of the cilia propel it back to the nostrils to be expelled, or down towards the throat to be swallowed. (These cilia are destroyed by smoking a cigarette, and take ten days to grow back). In the nasal cavity, the temperature of the air begins to adjust to body temperature before entering the lungs.

The lining of the nose also contains chemoreceptors, specialised sensory neurons which detect chemicals in the air entering the nose, transmit this information via the olfactory nerve to the brain, where it is registered as smell. The term for this process is olfaction.

The pharynx is the common channel for both food and air at the back of the mouth, where there is a small flap of tissue called the epiglottis. The epiglottis acts as a valve to regulate the flow of air to and from the larynx and food into the oesophagus, the tube connecting the mouth and stomach. Food or drink can sometimes go down the wrong way; coughing and sneezing are attempts to throw it back up. The tonsils, patches of lymphoid tissue, are attached to the wall of the pharynx, where they can trap and destroy foreign particles entering the body in the air.

The larynx, which contains the voice box, is made of cartilage joined by ligaments and membranes. Folds of tissue in the voice box vibrate and make a sound when air passes over them. A man's larynx is larger than a

Figure 8: The structure of the respiratory system.

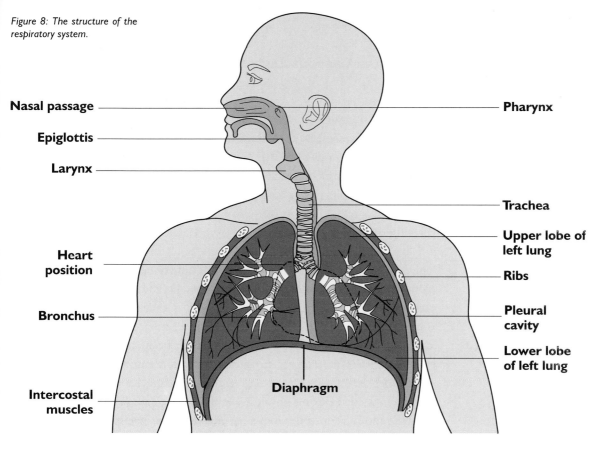

Nasal passage

Epiglottis

Larynx

Heart position

Bronchus

Intercostal muscles

Pharynx

Trachea

Upper lobe of left lung

Ribs

Pleural cavity

Lower lobe of left lung

Diaphragm

woman's, and is commonly called an Adam's apple.

The trachea, commonly known as the windpipe, can be felt easily at the front of the throat. It is a muscular tube reinforced by rings of cartilage. The oesophagus lies behind the trachea, and the thyroid and parathyroid glands are wrapped around the trachea at the level of the larynx.

The lungs, two sacs of smooth muscle, lie in the thoracic cavity, either side of the heart, extending from just under the clavicles to the diaphragm. Each is divided into lobes; the right lung has three, and the left two, there being less room in the left side of the chest due to the position of the heart. The lungs are covered with pleural membrane, which also lines the inside of the entire thoracic cavity. These pleura secrete a fluid to lubricate the tissues, and ease movement of the lungs against the ribs.

Just below the junction of the clavicles and sternum, the trachea divides into two tubes, also ringed in cartilage, called the bronchi. On entering the lungs, each bronchus divides into smaller and smaller tubes, with less cartilage and muscle, called bronchioles, which fill the lung, looking somewhat like the root system of a tree.

Alveoli and Gaseous Exchange

Each bronchiole ends in a little air sac, or alveolus, which is surrounded by a network of capillaries. The walls of the alveoli are elastic to allow for stretching and recoil as air enters the lungs and is expelled. They are also thin enough for gases to diffuse through into the capillaries and vice versa. Oxygen from the air breathed in diffuses through the alveolar wall into the blood in the capillaries, where it combines with haemoglobin, a chemical in red blood cells, to form oxyhaemoglobin. Blood that contains red cells carrying oxygen in this way is called oxygenated blood.

The capillaries around the alveolus also contain blood entering the lungs from the body, with the waste gas, carbon dioxide, dissolved in it. Blood containing carbon dioxide and not oxygen is called deoxygenated blood. Carbon dioxide diffuses from the blood in the capillaries through the alveolar wall into the alveolus, and leaves the body as air is expelled. This two way process is called gaseous exchange. The rate of gaseous exchange determines levels of oxygen and carbon dioxide in the body. If more oxygen is needed during physical exertion, for example, we breathe faster, to bring more air into the lungs. In this way, the respiratory system has a homeostatic function.

Inside each lung, the capillaries that like the bronchioles form a system looking like a tree root, link up into two vessels, the pulmonary vein, which carries oxygenated blood from the lung to the heart, and the pulmonary artery, which brings deoxygenated blood from the heart into the lung.

Note: The pulmonary veins are the only veins in the body to carry oxygenated blood; all other veins bring deoxygenated blood from the tissues to the heart. The pulmonary arteries are the only arteries in the body to carry deoxygenated blood; all other arteries carry oxygenated blood away from the heart.

The heart, made of specialised muscle called cardiac muscle, has its own built in pacemaker that initiates and maintains contraction. The sinoatrial node, in the wall of the right atrium, receives input from the vagus nerve, part of the parasympathetic nervous system, which maintains the resting heartbeat; usually 70 beats per minute in adults. Other nerves to the heart, the cardiac nerves, are innervated by sympathetic nervous system activity to increase heartrate.

The heart, being a constantly working muscle, also needs a good blood supply. The coronary blood vessels that encircle it arise from the first part of the aorta, bringing blood out of the heart and directly to the heart muscle.

Functions of the Heart

The heart's purpose is to pump blood from the body to the lungs for a fresh supply of oxygen, and then to pump this blood from the lungs to the rest of the body. Both atria contract together, then both ventricles contract together; there is a simultaneous shutting of the valves. Deoxygenated blood, i.e. blood that has circulated through the tissues and lost its oxygen supply, enters the right atrium, which contracts forcing the blood into the right ventricle and shutting the valves. The right ventricle contracts, forcing blood out into the pulmonary artery, which carries it to the lungs. Simultaneously, oxygenated blood from the lungs enters the left atrium, is forced into the left ventricle, then out into the aorta, the main artery in the body.

Circulation of the Blood

Within the whole circulation system there are some sub-circuits which have particular functions:

1. The systemic circulation. This is the circuit that carries blood from the heart in the aorta, through a network of finer and finer vessels to all the cells in the body, and returns it to the heart in the inferior vena cava from the lower body or the superior vena cava from the upper body.
2. The pulmonary circulation. The circuit that transports blood from the heart to the lungs and back again is called the pulmonary circulation.
3. The hepatic portal system. Blood from the small intestines carrying the products of digestion, is taken to the liver before being returned to the venous system for return to the heart. This detour is to enable nutrients and toxins to be removed from the blood for storage or destruction in the liver.

Blood Vessels

All blood vessels are hollow tubes forming the pipework of the system. The walls have an outer layer of connective tissue, a middle layer of smooth muscle, and an inner layer of epidermal tissue. Expansion of the central cavity is called vasodilation; when it contracts it is called vasoconstriction.

Arteries are the vessels that carry blood away from the heart. (A tip to remember: arteries and away both begin with a). The smooth muscle layer is much thicker than in the other blood vessels, because these vessels need to expand and withstand the pressure of blood as it is pumped from the heart. The recoil of the muscular walls also helps to propel blood along. If an artery is damaged, a lot of blood can be very quickly lost, often with fatal results. Hence, they tend to be in the safest areas of the limbs to minimise this risk – passing on the inside of joints as in the armpit, elbow, wrist, or back of the knee, often together with the nerves which are similarly protected. They also tend to be deep in the body, except for a very few places; in the wrist and throat the pulse can be easily felt in the radial or carotid artery respectively. The largest artery leading out of the heart is the aorta. As they branch out into the tissues, arteries become smaller in diameter, and are called arterioles.

Apart from the pulmonary artery going to the lungs, all of the arteries in the body carry oxygenated blood.

The vessels continue to decrease in size until they become capillary networks. These are found in all tissues with the exception of the epidermis of the skin, hair and nails. Some tissues, such as skeletal muscle, have very extensive capillary networks; others, like connective tissue, have very little. Capillaries are very thin walled vessels, so thin that they are permeable, and the nutrients, hormones, antibodies and other large molecules in the blood, as well as white blood cells, can pass through into the intercellular fluid, and waste material can pass into the capillaries.

As it begins its journey back to the heart, blood passes first into venules then into the similar but larger veins. Veins have thinner walls than the arteries, and another important feature; one way valves. As the blood passes through, the valves shut to prevent the back flow. Blood moves much more slowly back towards the heart; there is no force to pump it back and often it is working against the pull of gravity. So what moves it?

Figure 9: The blood vessels of the head and neck.

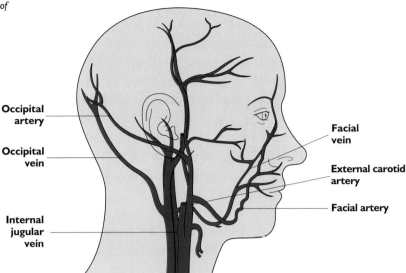

Occipital artery

Occipital vein

Internal jugular vein

Facial vein

External carotid artery

Facial artery

To some extent, it is pulled back by suction, as blood empties from the two venae cavae into the heart. Another important factor, especially in the legs, is the effect of muscles squeezing the blood vessels as they contract for action, thereby pumping blood back through the veins. Unlike arteries, veins are often close to the surface in the limbs, which is why heavy massage strokes that squeeze the muscles need to be done 'towards the heart' when working on the limbs.

The Lymphatic System

In the capillary networks, the fluid part of the blood, plasma, filters through into the tissues, becoming intercellular fluid. Not all of this is reabsorbed into the capillaries. The rest is picked up by the lymphatic ducts and returned to the blood supply in the subclavian veins, under the clavicles, having been filtered through the lymph nodes. Flow of lymph, like venous blood, depends on suction and muscle pumping.

Blood

Blood consists of 55% liquid plasma and 45% blood cells and materials dissolved in the water, which are being transported round the body. Plasma is a straw-coloured liquid that is composed of water, minerals, proteins, hormones, waste which includes urea, and nutrients.

The precursors of all blood cells are made in red bone marrow, and differentiate into three main groups.

Red blood cells, or erythrocytes, give the blood its colour. They are biconcave and are unusual in having no nucleus. Their function is to transport oxygen around the body from the lungs; in the alveoli, oxygen attaches to a chemical called haemoglobin in the erythrocyte. Once it reaches the tissues, oxygen is released for use in cell metabolism. Erythrocytes have a life span of about 120 days and are destroyed in the liver or spleen.

Leucocytes, or white blood cells, are all involved in defending the body. They live for a few hours to a few days and have the ability to change shape, leave the blood by squeezing out of capillary walls, and to migrate through the tissues.

There are five different kinds: neutrophils and monocytes are able to engulf and destroy bacteria, viruses and foreign material through a process called phagocytosis. Monocytes are called macrophages when in the tissues rather than the circulation; the lymph nodes are full of macrophages. Easinophils and basophils are the white cells involved in allergic responses, and lymphocytes, which include T cells and B cells, are involved in the adaptive immune response.

Platelets are small cells that are responsible for clotting blood. When exposed to air or objects that have penetrated the blood vessel, they stick together to plug the hole in the vessel wall, and combine with one of the proteins in the plasma, fibrinogen, to form a clot. The latter process is called coagulation.

Massage Considerations

In healthy people, there are two considerations for massage relating to the cardiovascular system:

1. Never put heavy or prolonged pressure on the major superficial arteries. These are the two arteries where you feel for a pulse, the carotid at the side of the neck and the ulnar on the inner surface of the wrist, and the arteries on the inner surface of the elbow joint, and the back of the knee.

2. When massaging the limbs with firm pressure, work towards the heart. If you massage firmly in the opposite direction, there is a danger of turning the valves in the veins inside out and permanently damaging them.

Part 4
The Practice of Indian Head Massage

The Chakra (Spinning Wheel of Energy) System

In the West, we have little time to pursue spiritual development and even our personal time is limited. Therefore, our spiritual growth is not prioritised as much as one would like or even believe to exist. The first law of nature in our learning and development is 'self-preservation'. Therefore, our foundation is linked to our physical, mental and emotional wellbeing, something we very often ignore or do not respect enough. By focusing in and around us, we can begin to balance ourselves in our world and achieve focus, clarity and vision within our own lives.

Just as our diet and nutrition is the key to helping maintain our physical selves, spiritual development is the key to the maintenance of our mental and emotional wellbeing. One way of developing our spiritual side is through the balance of our Chakra System.

There are many understandings and versions of this concept; ours is a simple understanding. The Chakra is an ancient Sanskrit word which means a 'spinning wheel of energy' that vibrates and controls physical and psychic energy. There are many points of the Chakra in and around the body. In Indian Head Massage, we focus on the major seven points passing through the body. The Chakra System is closely linked to the endocrine and nervous systems of the human body. Various chemical

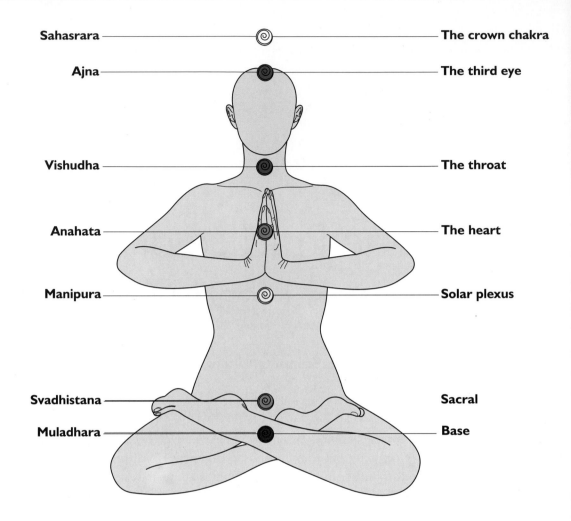

Sahasrara ———————————————— The crown chakra

Ajna ———————————————— The third eye

Vishudha ———————————————— The throat

Anahata ———————————————— The heart

Manipura ———————————————— Solar plexus

Svadhistana ———————————————— Sacral

Muladhara ———————————————— Base

reactions are influenced by our Chakra System such as the releasing of seratonin which can bring on the feel good factor, once massage is introduced. Our Chakra System is activated at birth after leaving the mother's body, which has so far been dormant whilst within the womb. Our physical and intuitive nature is responding to the energies around us, Earth's energy being penetrated through the feet and the Universal energy through the crown of the head.

The seven major Chakras are as follows with Eastern names and corresponding parts of the physical, mental and emotional:

Please note that these are very basic interpretations of the whole Chakra System. There is much more depth to this subject incorporating the subconscious and energies on a higher plane.

Sanskrit Name	Colour	Representation
Sahasrara	White	**The Crown Chakra** – The brain and pineal gland relating to Universal energies.
Ajna	Indigo	**The Third Eye Chakra** – Centre of the forehead, part of the lower brain, the pituitary gland and the nervous system. Opening up of psychic and intuitive awareness.
Vishudha	Blue	**The Throat Chakra** – The thyroid, throat and all parts of the vocal system. The communication area which relates to your oral speech and sounds. One of the physical self-expressions.
Anahata	Green	**The Heart Chakra** – Around the centre of the chest. The heart, thymus and circulatory system. The soul system where we initiate our 'intuitive reactions', from where our emotion is affected.
Manipura	Yellow	**The Solar Plexus Chakra** – Around the top of the stomach and diaphragm area, also affecting the nervous system, stomach and liver. The centre of your being where we connect with Universal and Earthly energies as one. Your foundation which can develop your unique spirituality. Where the first law of nature begins 'self-preservation'.
Svadhistana	Orange	**The Sacral Chakra** – The reproductive system, ovaries and testes. Just one of our many experiences of nature. The beginning of the physical life.
Muladhara	Red	**The Base Chakra** – The peroneum, the foundation of the physical. The human beings most intimate and possible personal connection.

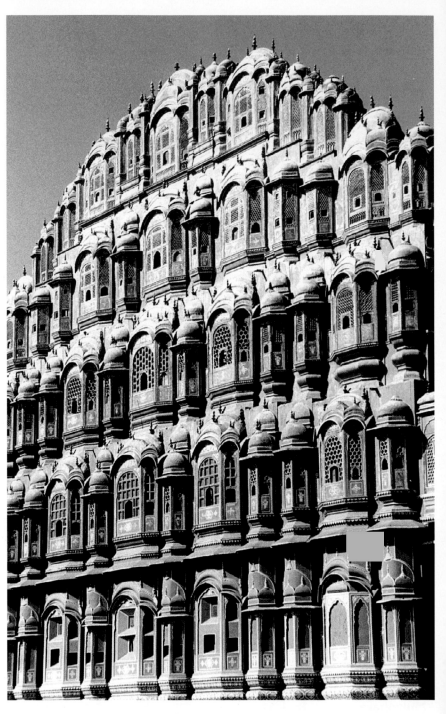

Although we talk about the spiritual development and we deal with indefinable energies, remember that we must be earthed at all times and not let ourselves to be drawn into false existence which can manipulate our lives, causing painful relationships with ourselves and others.

How Does it Relate to Indian Head Massage?

As human beings, we are all part of the big picture, the Universe. When we fall ill, it is because we have somehow disconnected ourselves from the universal force. We are all sustained by the universal force through specifically chosen vortices of energy attached through the body known as 'Chakras'.

As well as concentrating on the physical, we are also alerting the mental and emotional aspects, and for this we are working on and with the Universal or Spiritual energies. This then focuses on the Chakra System and helps open up theses vortices of energy, which may be laid dormant or not as effective as they should be, causing mental, emotional, and physical blockages.

The experience of this is a very personal one and clients can often relate to it best through the colours they experience around the Ajna (third eye). There should be no fear, but a reassurance of the clarity needed to define the problematic area whether physically, mentally or emotionally. 'Focus, Clarity and Vision'!

As well as the massage, we can also balance Chakras for others, using a very simple process which includes a gentle healing process:

- Ask the recipient to sit or lay down.
- Using a pendant or crystal on a chain, hold about 15cms away from the Chakra point.
- Place one hand at the back of the body at least 15cms away.
- Without any movement from yourself, the pendant will start to spin. This is when the Chakra is being balanced.
- A stagnating pendant will indicate a block of energy. It is then that the therapist would need to work with the client to unblock the vortices of energy.

This is a very simple, yet effective process. However, make sure that the recipient understands the concept of Chakra balancing before you begin; any fear of the unknown can slow down the process. The whole concept of Chakra balancing is applied and delivered using unconditional energy. So as much as we may want to help the recipient, if we put conditions on the subject, it will prevent the required faith of the unknown positive energy.

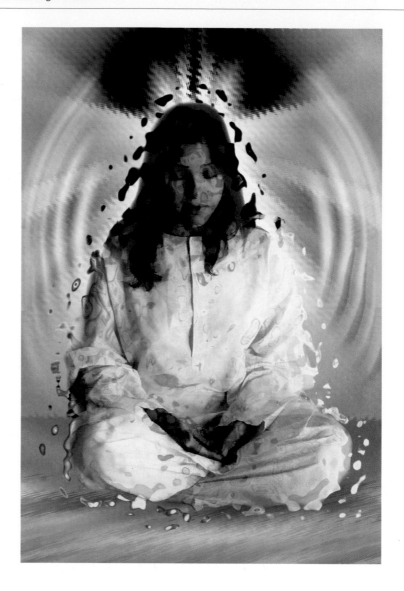

The Therapeutic Value of Sound and Music Within Treatment

Sound and music is part of everyday life. It exists at the beginning and end of each new day, yet changes subtly in meaning all the time. Our own interpretation can turn any sound into music and our general mental and physical state can cope with certain sounds at certain times. Sound and music also trigger memories with times of contentment or challenges, our subconscious is alerted and a process of visualisation begins, to which we may react. It is therefore a very personal experience and we are able to bring to it our own ideas and beliefs in times when it is in our control.

Even to those who suffer with the loss of hearing, there are sounds within the head or pulses which play a rhythm. Sound is one of the most common forms of entertainment used today. It can work for a collective or singular audience, yet it carries very different meanings. We very often turn to music for calm, stimulation, escape or just noise, so the feeling of loneliness is abated. Music has great control of our emotions and can manipulate feelings such as empathy in individuals. Look at how film makers use music to enhance our feelings of empathy at emotional junctures of the story.

In ancient times, music was used by people as a form of communication within religion. When a collective made music through singing and praying, it caused a bond which the people could relate to and where common ground was felt.

Within Yoga, there are several physical positions which can, along with our control of breathing, alter our heart rate to modify our function. Music is one of the tools which can be used to alter our perceptions and therefore manipulate our body structure for reaction.

Depending on the type of music we listen to, an appreciation of harmonious and calming music has a beautiful positive effect on the body. Even if we do not recognise this physically, mentally and emotionally, it can override our moods and state of mind.

When we listen to a certain melody, it is quite easy to manipulate ourselves to think happy contented thoughts, sometimes very simple yet effective. This stimulus can in effect slow the physical body down to release the tensions out of the muscles, giving us the ability to function effectively and improve our state of consciousness. It can evoke the focus, clarity and vision attained during our meditative state.

How Does it Work for Indian Head Massage?

Apart from being enjoyable and bringing a certain mystique to the treatment, it does have other qualities. This all depends on the type of music used and it must be fitting for the scenario that you have created.

- By using a particular piece of music which is repetitive and has a slower beat, we can achieve a more peaceful and relaxed treatment.
- Some studies have also shown that relaxing gentle music has the

ability to reduce headaches, lower your anxiety levels and steady the heart rate which can bring down the stress and tension.

- On a more universal note, with the repetitive sound, the music eases the subconscious therefore relaxing deeper and bringing a focus and clarity to the conscious mind. An inner communication is achieved leaving the client transported through the hypnotic effect of sound/music and touch.
- Above all, the mind clears and one can begin rational thinking into life's challenges.

It is true to say that the combination of music and a therapeutic massage work hand in hand. However, there may be clients who are irritated by your choice of music, so find a happy medium which pleases both parties as this is also a medium for the therapist.

Once we become well-trained and competent in Indian Head Massage, our own goals may shift and we may enter another phase of development where all our movements and actions are slower and taken with unconditional energies. We too are transported by the physical and psychological massage, through music and touch.

A rejuvenation process can occur for client and therapist, and at this stage we realise that we are well on our way to achieving our goals and ambitions for a life above and beyond our conscious limitations.

Colouring Breaths

1. Breathe into your body the colour red twice, then imagine being surrounded by the colour red.
2. Breathe in orange, then imagine being surrounded by the colour.
3. Breathe in yellow, then imagine being surrounded by the colour.
4. Breathe in green, then imagine being surrounded by the colour.
5. Breathe in blue, then imagine being surrounded by the colour.
6. Breathe in indigo, then imagine being surrounded by the colour.
7. Breathe in white, then imagine being surrounded by the colour.

Once you have completed the cycle gently, make sure that you are aware of your surroundings and then begin to open your eyes slowly. You have now completely energised your body. Drink a glass of water and take some time to reflect on how you feel.

Continuing this meditation will act as a self-help programme for you in times of extreme stress and tension. The more you do, the easier and more effective it becomes.

Time is not always on our side and sometimes our concentration for the colours can be poor, as day to day stresses inevitably encroach upon the meditation. On these occasions, even taking a minute to practice deep breathing in and out as a form of relaxation before beginning a treatment or facing any challenge through the day. This can create a feeling of calm and balance.

Routines to Relieve Stress and Tension – Short Techniques

As considered earlier, before we focus on releasing other peoples' stresses and tensions, we may want to focus on our own. Listed in this book are some self-help techniques to bring calm and balance to oneself through the gentle meditation.

There are many considerations to be made before applying any form of therapeutic treatment; the consultation for medical history, the perceptions of the client's personality and the treatment itself. However, we have researched some very simple yet effective techniques which you can use without going into too much detail.

We firstly need to know that the person receiving treatment is in generally good shape. Then we may assure the person of gentle pressures that we may use. Again we look to an aesthetically pleasing room, warm, quiet, not too bright and possibly a gentle sound of relaxation music.

Ask the recipient to sit in an upright chair, with their eyes closed having taken several deep breaths. The giver also begins with deep breaths and warm hands. We can now begin.

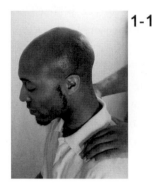 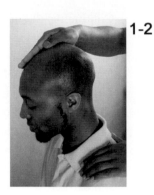

1. Place both hands on the shoulders one at a time, gently and slowly, then wait until you begin to feel a warmth or tingling sensation.

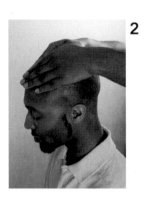

2. Place both hands on top of the head one at a time, gently and slowly, then wait until you begin to feel a warmth or tingling sensation.

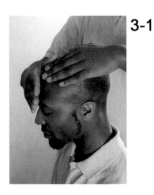 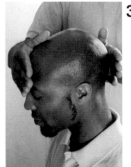

3. Place one hand on the forehead and the other hand on the back of the head, then wait until you begin to feel a warmth or tingling sensation.

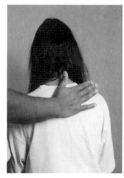
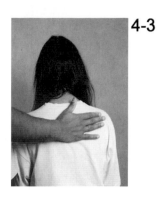
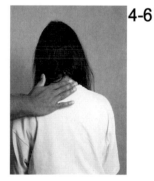

4. Place one hand on the shoulder and with the palm of the other hand, rub gently in anti-clockwise circles.

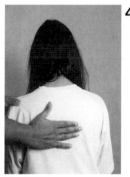
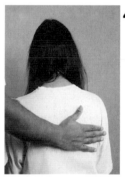
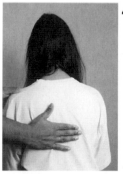

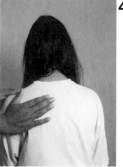
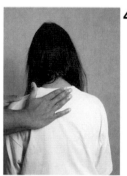

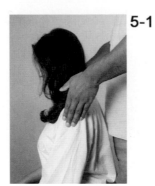 5-1

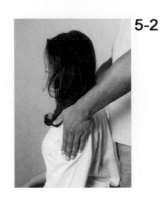 5-2

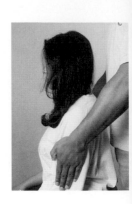

5. Smooth down the arms three times, bringing the hands up from the back.

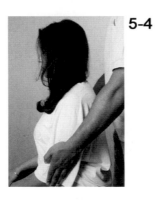 5-4

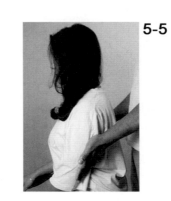 5-5

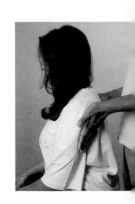

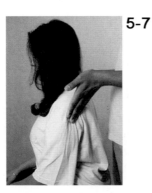 5-7

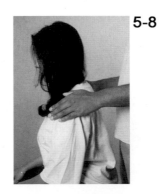 5-8

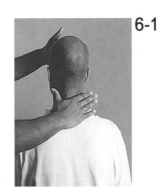

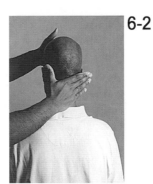

6. Place one hand on the forehead and begin to stroke the neck upwardly using very gentle strokes slowly.

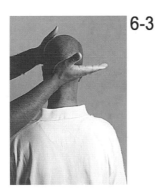

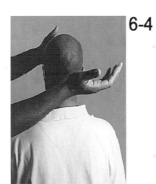

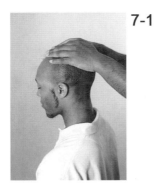

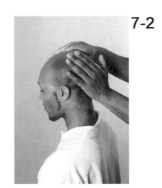

7. Place both hands on the top of the head and begin to stroke the head, using one hand after the other.

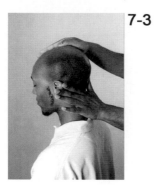

7-3

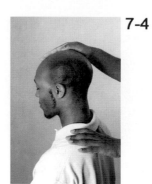

7-4

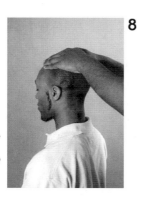

8

8. Return both hands to the top of the head and hold there for a short while, take a deep breath and then wait until you begin to feel a warmth or tingling sensation.

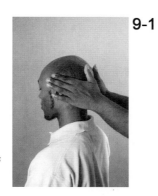

9-1

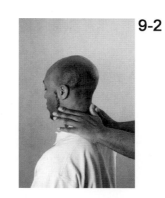

9-2

9. Finally glide both hands to the shoulders and release gently away.

This is a simple and effective way of introducing the full therapeutic massage. A complete version should be taught by a professional qualified teacher/trainer who has had at least five years' experience in the field.

Please note this is not the treatment used by professionals and should be restricted to friends and family.

As stated earlier in the book, the application of paste or cream can have a surprisingly profound effect to create good feelings and a 'natural high'. The best is probably a sandalwood paste which is commonly used in India before meditation. Sandalwood paste can be bought in select shops or can easily be made at home by rubbing the sandalwood in a pestle and mortar and adding a few drops of water and pinches of organic camphor and saffron. The paste can be used in massage over the forehead, eyebrows and temples.

A Guide to Sensual Massage – The Effects of Touch

Touch is undoubtedly one of the most important forms of communication known today. It is used everyday in all aspects of our lives and holds the key to many of the problems in our lives. There is a large population around the world that is starved of this form of communication, often older people, and it seems to be getting worse as the more technical and inventive sides to our world progresses.

The communication of touch is a fundamental medium for massage and must be delivered with compassion, otherwise we are delivering merely mechanical movements which have little effect. Applying harsh touch can even be counterproductive, causing the body to defend itself and rendering the technique ineffective. This could cause mental, physical, and sometimes emotional distress. With effective touch we are stimulating the nervous system and promoting mental, social and physical development. This healthy communication leads to a sense of comfort and compassion.

Touch through massage can also be a very sensual form of communication. This is mostly seen in couples, as partners wish to show their emotional feelings through physical means. The sensual touch shown by adults to one another is very different to the caring touch shown for children or as an unconditional feeling.

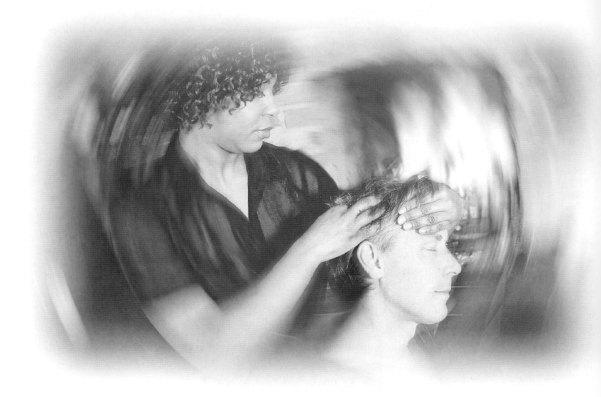

We link back again to the ancient times of the Karma Sutra, when a set of explicit illustrations were drawn to promote the art of physical love through sensual touch. It is a very natural, yet private suggestion and bonds two people together. Very often we have an overwhelming sense of affection and emotion that sweeps across our mind and body which is neither rational, or controlled. This is the 'moment' that sensual touch through massage can heighten your senses and develop a oneness with mind, body and soul.

Performing Indian Head Massage for Partners as a Theme for Sensual Touch

Allow an uninterrupted amount of time to fulfil each other's needs, with a time for sleep afterwards. This is preferably done after sunset.

'The Setting'

An aesthetically pleasing room – warm, soft lighting, possibly candles. The burning of a relaxing oil, accompanied by gentle flowing music.

'The Attire'

The massage you apply will still be performed over clothing – loosely fitting clothing which will cause no restrictions, i.e. soft or silky to the touch. Clothing restrictions are lifted once the massage is complete!

'The Massage'

This massage is performed in total harmony of all the senses:

- Both parties must close their eyes and follow a gentle breathing pattern to start.
- No verbal communication is allowed.
- The touch is soft and very gentle, barely touching.
- All strokes are gently flowing to the rhythm of the music and breathing.
- Pay particular attention to the neck and the ears.

Obviously everybody has their own interpretations of sensuality and its uniqueness in their lives. It is a very powerful tool for bonding and reconciliation. Have fun and enjoy the pleasures in paradise!

Oil Scalp Massage – Eastern and Western Approaches

Eastern Oil Scalp Massage

Oil applied to the head is absorbed into the roots of the hair, which, in turn, are connected with nerve fibres leading directly to the brain. Oil strengthens the hair and removes dryness which is responsible for brittle hair and for so many scalp disorders. By relaxing muscles and nerves, fatigue is eliminated from the system.

Oil to Use for Head Massage

Sesame seed oil extracted from black sesame seeds is supposed to be the best for hair. Sesame seed oil alone may be used, or mustard seed oil alone may be used by males. Coconut oil may be used by females. There are more oils which are beneficial for head massage:

- Amla oil.
- Bhringrag oil.
- Brahmi Amla oil.
- Brahmi Amla Shikekai.
- Brahmi Amla Bhringraj Shikekai.
- Sesame seed oil plus Almond oil plus Sandalwood oil.
- Sesame seed oil plus Almond oil plus Jasmin oil.
- Sesame seed oil plus Almond oil.
- Pumpkin seed oil.
- Kahu oil.
- Coriander oil.
- Mixture of Kahu plus Pumpkin seed oil plus Almond oil.

The masseur should make the subject sit down in a comfortable position. Then ask the subject to measure the first point, by measuring eight finger widths above the eyebrows, put his finger on the spot – and pour the oil. No patting or kneading is done on the head, as it is done on the other parts of the body. Massage starts after pouring the oil. The oil is uniformly distributed by the fingers of both the hands of the masseur by rubbing from the spot simultaneously towards the sides of the skull up to the temples. Then oil is poured at the second spot, and oil is again uniformly distributed by the fingers towards the side. Finally, oil is poured on the third spot, and the oil is again distributed by the same method of using all the fingers (*see* page 23 for the specific location of the spots).

- Press the point on the medulla oblongata, then bring the fingers towards the forehead along the sides of both ears.
- Then pound the head with the hand joints loosely together to excite the fine capillaries of the circulatory system and the nervous system.
- Next, rub the important spots as shown in the illustrations, with the hairs being twisted at the cowlick and the tenth gate.
- After this, press the skull with both the hands, with a little additional pressure.
- Before doing the massage of the face and the forehead, the hairs are twisted on all three spots – and then pulled gently.
- Then starts the massage of the forehead from the mind. The point on the eyebrows is the location of the second Chakra. The head massage ends after doing the face massage.
- The masseur should rub their fingers gently on the scalp – and pull the hairs on the top of the cranium; the location of the first Chakra – and clap.

- If one wants better results with the massage, a drop of oil should be poured into each ear. The subject should move his lower jaws to allow the oil to go deeper inside the ear. Also a drop of rose water should be dropped into the eyes.

Shiro-Abhyang (Head Massage) Technique

The head is the vital organ consisting of controlling centres of all the sense organs. It is the most important 'Marma'. Head massage relieves all 'Shirorogas' (it includes all types of headache arising from different causes). Head massage relieves itching and dryness of scalp.

Moordh Taila describes the process by which oil is applied to the head by various methods for a specific period.

Uses:

- Prevents headache.
- Prevents falling and greying of hair.
- Gives sound sleep.
- Makes hair long and beautiful.

There are four types/methods, which are progressively more and more effective; Shiro-Abhyang, Shirodhara, Shiropichu and Shirobasti respectively. The most common of these being the Shirodhara outlined below (this should last for $1/2$-1 hour).

Instruments used:

- Dharapatra (vessel) with a chain.
- A stand to which the chain is attached.
- A table.
- Oil/ghee/buttermilk.
- Cotton pads to cover the eyes.

Procedure

The room should be a calm and quiet place. For the constitution of Vata Dosha, oil/ghee should be lukewarm. For the constitution of Pitta, a material should be of room temperature.

The patient is advised to lie down on the table. Two small cotton pads dipped in rose water are placed on the eyes. Oil/ghee is poured over the forehead at a point just above the midpoint of the eyebrows. It is done from the height of about four fingers. The drip should not be too slow or too fast.

It is strictly to be done in the morning. After Shirodhara, medicated ghee is given orally according to the disease. Exertion is avoided.

Uses:

- Increases memory.
- Gives stability of mind.
- Gives sound sleep.
- Reduces body heat.

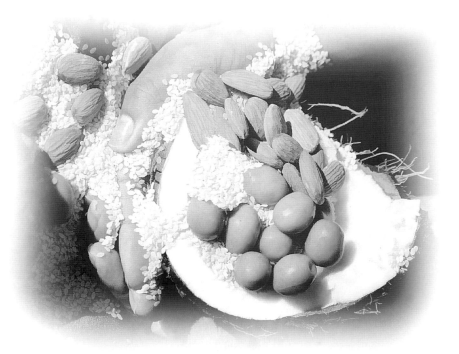

Indian Head Massage and Carrier Oils

Indian Head Massage is one of the most relaxing and mind-blowing experiences. With its many physical, physiological and mental effects on the body and mind, its benefits can be increased with the use of carrier oils. Indian Head Massage is an excellent opportunity to introduce a carrier to stimulate hair growth, improve scalp condition and ameliorate (improve) skin problems. This section will help practitioners of Indian Head Massage to increase the benefits of this treatment.

Use of Carrier Oils in Indian Head Massage

The therapist's choice of carrier oils for head massage must be governed by their applicability. It is the characteristics of the medium which will determine which carrier oil is best to use.

Carrier oils can enhance the treatment and add to its valuable quality in the resulting outcome. They can promote healing, speed up expulsion of toxins, nourish the scalp and the hair follicles, relax and enhance the treatment by providing emollient to prevent friction. They increase the beneficial effects of this treatment.

As an added bonus, 'fixed oils' can enrich the body systems by supplying vitamins and minerals which can contribute positively to the general health of the recipient.

The four carrier oils described in this section have been carefully chosen. They are easily available on the market, they are not too greasy, and their properties can dramatically enhance Indian Head Massage treatment.

In many geographical areas of the world, the coconut and mustard seed oils are used traditionally in the head and scalp massage. Coconut oil is used in the Caribbean Islands and mustard seed oil is very popular in India, Nepal and Pakistan. However, in Europe, the sweet almond oil and the sesame seed oil are commonly used in body massage.

The carrier oils need to be carefully checked for quality – the cold pressed and unrefined oils are the best. Although they may be higher in price, the success of the treatment may outweigh financial expense.

We need only a small amount of carrier oil for treatment – enough to be spread over the area of both palms of the practitioner's hands, and then treatment can start. More carrier oil may be needed for long hair. This may be applied before the start of the treatment by running the fingers through the hair strands in a slow and rhythmical fashion – caressing rather than pulling. This technique of application allows the recipient to become accustomed to the practitioner's way of handling the hair. Gentle, slow, rhythmical and thorough movement of the hands is very soothing and extremely relaxing. Therefore, the outcome of this approach will be equally relaxing and beneficial.

Fixed oils do not evaporate. They are plant oils used as an emollient to either prevent friction during massage or to facilitate absorption of pure essential oils. Cold pressed and unrefined carrier oils retain properties of the original raw material content of vitamins and trace elements. They leave a greasy mark on paper. They are not soluble in alcohol and they are not miscible with water. They do, on the other hand, mix with chloroform, ether and petroleum spirit.

Natural, as opposed to synthetic, fixed oils consist of natural lipids, esters and triacylglycerols. They are usually referred to as vegetable oils which, if extracted by a cold-pressed technique, are unrefined and from organic material. They form a 'living' matter which can enrich Indian Head Massage treatment.

Sweet Almond Oil

Sweet almond oil (*Prunus dulcis, P amygdalis var.dulcis*) originates from the Rosaceae family.

Prunus in Latin means 'plum tree', dulcis means 'sweet' and amygdalis, (Greek amugdale and Latin amygdalis) are names for the plant.

The almond tree has been known and cultivated for thousands of years in the Middle East region and the Mediterranean countries. Greek and Italian traders introduced almonds to Europe. The tree is quite small in height and its fruits are of light green colour and a 'furry' outer skin.

Sweet almond oil is one of the most popular oils used in pharmacy and as a carrier oil in tactile treatments such as the Indian Head Massage, body massage and aromatherapy. The oil is pale yellow in colour. Sweet almond oil is viscous hence its absorption through the skin is slower and the oil should be warmed before treatment. Higher temperature aids less viscosity and it is recommended that therapists warm their hands before treatment. When the oil is applied with warm hands and on a warm skin, its penetration is increased. Sweet almond oil can keep for a long time without going rancid if it is stored correctly in an airtight container, a dark cupboard and at a cool temperature.

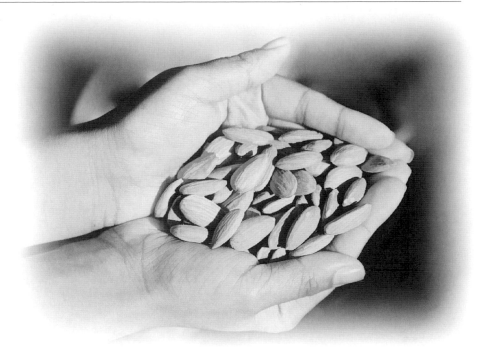

The popularity of sweet almond oil among body workers is due to the fact that it has a delicate sweet smell and contains Vitamins A, B1, B2, B6, and Vitamin E. It is considered beneficial in the treatment of skin inflammation and the itching of dry, chapped skin. Its emollient properties render this oil very effective in the treatment of psoriasis and dermatitis. Sweet almond oil is suitable for treatment in Indian Head Massage if the scalp is dry and hair is brittle and breaking easily.

For a greasy scalp and overproduction from the sebaceous glands, Indian Head Massage treatment should include sweet almond oil with a touch of lemongrass. The scalp should become stabilised after a few intensive treatments and clients can be prescribed a hair/scalp massage oil of lemongrass in a carrier of sweet almond oil to use at home on a daily basis. However:

*   Some people are allergic to almond nuts and although sweet almond oil has been found non-irritating to rabbit skin in its 25% solution, therapists are advised to check for allergies before applying this oil in Indian Head Massage.
*   The oil of bitter almond is not used in body massage due to its toxic content of hydrocyanic acid (prussic acid). Bitter almond essential oil free from prussic acid has its culinary uses and is also used in the food industry.

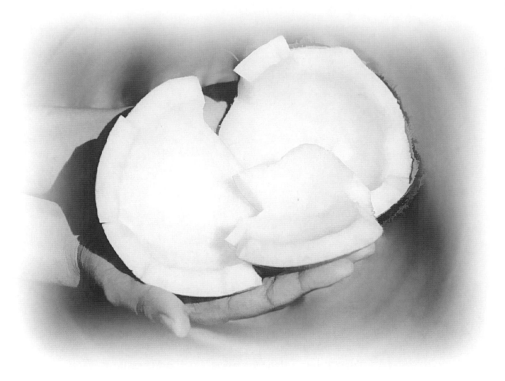

Coconut Oil

The choice of this oil for application in hair treatment is obvious. Coconut oil has been used for centuries in hair and skin care in geographical areas of Malaysia, Polynesia and the Caribbean Islands.

Coconut oil (*Cocos nucifera L*) originates from the Palmae family and it translates as 'monkey face'. It was believed that the shape of coconut (when cut) reminded indigenous people of a monkey face. The word nucifera translates as, 'bearing nuts'.

The palm tree grows to a height of 80 feet (25 metres). The fruit is a valuable commercial material and is cultivated in many tropical areas such as the African continent and Southeast Asia. The commercial part of the coconut is a hard endocarp and the seed. The 'milk' is the albumin of the seed, and a solid copra contains about 65% lipids.

The fully grown coconut tree – it reaches maturity after 30 years – can produce 80 coconuts per annum. However, some varieties of coconut trees on man-made plantations can yield up to 180–200 nuts per year.

Coconut oil is a white solid. This saturated fat has a melting temperature of 25°C. It is usually solid at room temperature, but may liquidise on a warm body and in the therapist's warm hands.

In Ayurvedic medicine, coconut oil is used in the treatment of burns, heart and circulatory problems. Its most pronounced action is in hair care treatment. It adds lustre to the hair. The shine of hair treated with coconut oil is healthy and attractive. Externally, coconut oil is frequently used in massage preparations because of its emollient characteristics.

Its prime cosmetic use is in hair care (a hair pomade), also in lipsticks and the production of soap. Many hair conditioners include coconut oil, as it is very beneficial for dry hair. In some tropical countries, people believe that the use of coconut oil in hair care every day, prevents greying and baldness.

However, Coconut oil may induce an allergic reaction of the skin in some people. This refers particularly to solvent extracted oil. Therapists are advised to check the quality of the product before use.

Sesame Seed Oil

One other popular fixed oil, which can be very useful in the treatment of Indian Head Massage, is sesame seed oil.

Sesame seed oil (Sesamum indicum DC) belongs to the Pedaliaceae family. Its name derives from the Egyptian 'semsemt'. The Egyptian papyrus mentions sesame in 1800 BC. Sesame relates to the God of the dead in Hindu religion.

The sesame plant, cultivated for at least 4000 years in Mesopotamia and found in the tomb of the Tutankhamun (1300 BC) boasts bell-shaped white flowers. The white seeds produce a superior quality oil, and black seeds are of a much lower commercial value.

Two natural antioxidants, sesamol and sesamolinol, are present in sesame seed oil, hence its rate of oxidisation is much lower than that of other carrier oils. Sesame seed oil is almost odourless and is high in vitamins A, B and E. It also contains certain minerals such as calcium, magnesium and phosphorus.

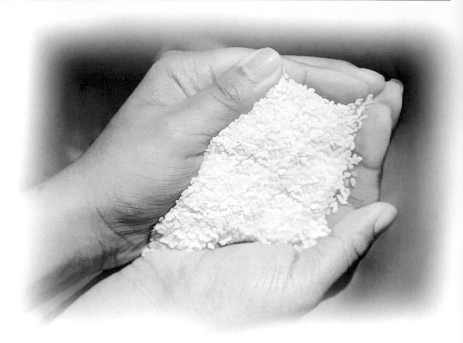

The oil has been traditionally used for disorders of the spleen and in cases of anaemia, particularly in children. It is high in calcium and when ingested, has a low acidity level. Sesame seed oil is an excellent massage medium in Indian Head Massage, particularly for clients with high blood cholesterol level.

Sesame seed oil lends itself to be used in Indian Head Massage because it soothes the skin of the scalp and counteracts dandruff. Also, it nourishes the hair follicles and encourages hair growth.

However, Sesame seed oil may cause hypersensitivity. It would be appropriate to test for skin sensitivity before employing this oil in Indian Head Massage treatment.

Mustard Seed Oil

The traditional use of mustard seed oil in skin and hair care in the Asian sub-continent prompted me to include this oil for use in Indian Head Massage.

Mustard seed oil (*Brassica nigra = Brassica sinapiodes = Sinapis nigra*) belongs to the Cruciferae family. The plant has pretty, bright flowers with a distinctive smell hidden within its seed. Mustard seed oil is extracted from black mustard seeds. It is a colourless to pale yellow liquid. Mustard

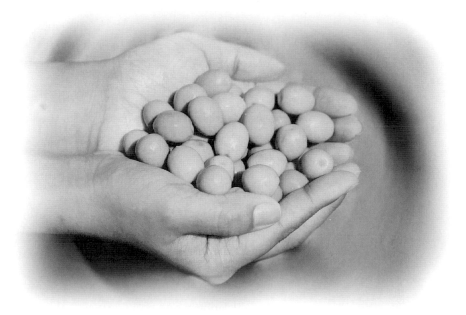

seed oil, obtained by pressing the seeds by mechanical means, does not contain allyl isothiocyanate. More advanced methods of extraction may even ameliorate its usual pungent and irritating smell.

Mustard seed oil has been used for centuries to prevent heart disease, blindness, bleeding duodenal ulcers and impotency. Nowadays, it is used for prevention of cancer, blood pressure, diabetes, arthritis and atherosclerosis. Mustard seed oil contains zinc (up to 5%) and magnesium (2.5%) although the mineral content does depend on the method of extraction.

In culinary application, mustard seed oil is very popular in cooking and spicy food preparations. Mustard itself contains no cholesterol, so it is very beneficial for people with a higher blood cholesterol level. Leaf mustard contains calcium, phosphorus, magnesium and Vitamin B.

The oil is believed to stimulate digestion. It can clear the sinuses and increases blood circulation (mustard plaster). Mustard seed oil is used for scalp and body massage as well as for hair care in many Asian countries. However,
- Mustard seed oil may irritate the skin.
- Although all the isothiocyanates found in their natural environment are considered toxic, the allyl isothiocyanate found in mustard seed

essential oil is the only one with a GRAS status. This is due to the fact that it has a strong anti-carcinogenic potential. The US National Cancer Institute plans to research it in the hope of finding preventative or even curative measures of cancer in humans and animals.

First Aid for the Therapist

Anyone, at any time, can feel unwell or have an accident. First aid is the immediate assistance given to that person from someone with appropriate training.

The Health and Safety at Work (First Aid) Regulations 1981, state that all employers have responsibilities to:

1.   Provide an appropriate level of first aid equipment for their staff.
2.   Provide appropriate training in first aid for staff members to act as first-aiders for other staff.
3.   Inform all employees of the arrangements made.

This law applies to all employers, of any size, including beauty and therapy salons. It is not a legal requirement for the self-employed therapist, as they do not have any employees working for them. However, in the interest of providing a complete and pleasant service for your clients, some knowledge of first aid is very useful.

It must be stressed at this point that the following information is just that – information. This section will consider the conditions most likely to confront a therapist:

- Fainting/feeling faint.
- Sprained joint.
- Bruising/swelling.
- Burns/scalds.
- Fractures/dislocations.
- Bleeding (including a nose bleed).
- Shock.
- Asthma.
- Anaphylactic shock.
- Epilepsy.
- Heart attack.

First Aid – Your Safety

Rule I

Never put yourself at risk to help someone else. In particular do not allow body fluids such as blood or vomit to come into contact with your skin.

Rule 2

Preserving life is your first priority. If you are not sure what to do, the best way to help is to get qualified medical assistance, usually by telephoning for the emergency services.

First Aid Conditions

Feeling Faint

Causes: Heat, illness, standing up too quickly after lying down.
Recognition: The casualty will look pale and feel dizzy.
Management: Sit the casualty down with their head between their knees.

Fainting

Causes: As above.
Recognition: The casualty will look pale and will become briefly unconscious.
Management: When the casualty regains consciousness, lie them flat, keep them warm and raise their feet about 15–30cms. This will help to keep more blood available for the head.

Sprained Joint

Causes: Twisting a joint, e.g. ankle, further than it is designed to go.
Recognition: Swelling, bruising, pain – especially when weight is put on the joint.
Management: **Rest.** Ask the casualty to sit and advise them not to drive.
                Ice. Anything cold, wrap it in a towel or bandage

before applying.

Compression. Apply a bandage if you have been trained.

Elevation. Raise the injured leg to help drain the fluids.

Always advise going to hospital for an X-ray as a precaution.

Bruising/swelling

Cause:	Any blow that does not break the skin, but causes bleeding underneath the skin.
Recognition:	Discolouration, swelling, pain.
Management:	Ice. Do not put in direct contact with the skin.

Fractures/dislocations

Causes:	A fall, or blow, that damages a bone or moves it out of place.
Recognition:	Pain, out of shape, a 'snap' may have been heard.
Management:	Do not move the casualty, but make them comfortable and get medical assistance.

Burns/scalds

Cause:	Contact with a hot object, fluid or steam.
Recognition:	Pain, redness, swelling, blistering.
Management:	Remove any wet clothing (unless it is stuck to the skin). Remove any watches and jewellery near the burnt area. Immerse in cold water, ideally a sink, with the tap running to keep it cold, for at least 10 minutes. Advise to seek medical attention.

Bleeding

Cause:	A sharp object cutting the skin or a blow to the nose.
Recognition:	Blood trickling/flowing from the wound or nose.
Management:	Ask the casualty to put pressure on the wound with their own hand. If it is a nose bleed, they should pinch the soft part of the nose and lean forward. Send them to get an appropriate level of medical assistance.

N.B. If the bleeding is very bad, telephone the emergency services.

Shock

Cause: Anyone who has been badly hurt will suffer from shock.

Recognition: Pale, clammy skin; shallow breathing; shivering; feel dizzy.

Management: If their injuries permit, lie them down, keep them warm and raise their legs 15–30cms.

Asthma

Cause: Dust, pollen, smoke, stress.

Recognition: Distressed, difficulty breathing, wheezing.

Management: Sit down, lean forward slightly; if they have medication, encourage them to take it but do not administer it yourself.

Anaphylactic Shock

Cause: Allergy to peanuts, insect stings and some other foodstuffs.

Recognition: The face will swell and go blotchy, breathing will become difficult and may stop.

Management: Telephone for the emergency services. If breathing stops and you have been trained, commence resuscitation.

Epilepsy

Cause: Triggered by many factors, including flickering lights.

Recognition: The most common form will cause the casualty to fall to the ground and their muscles to spasm uncontrollably.

Management   Do not touch or move the casualty. Remove any nearby objects that the casualty could injure themselves on and wait for the casualty to finish fitting. Advise them to seek medical advice, especially if they have never had a fit before or if they have bumped their head. If the fit lasts five minutes, or they have a second fit, telephone for the emergency services.

Heart Attack

Cause:	A blockage in an artery supplying the heart muscle.
Recognition:	Massive crushing pain in the chest, can spread to the left arm. The skin will be pale and clammy and breathing will be difficult.
Management:	Help the casualty into a comfortable position, usually a half-sitting position leaning against a wall or similar. Telephone for the emergency services.

The information given here is very basic but provides a few sensible rules. If these are followed, then these techniques are safe to use when necessary.

Rule 1	Ensure your own safety. Think danger!
Rule 2	If in doubt, get qualified help. Either a First Aider, or telephone for the emergency services.
Rule 3	Do not force the casualty to do anything they do not wish to do.
Rule 4	Do not administer any medications; that is the casualty's responsibility.

Appendix One

What is C.I.H.M.?

- C.I.H.M. stands for the Confederation of Indian Head Massage.
- C.I.H.M. is a professional body of lecturers/practitioners and students of Indian Head Massage.

What are the aims of C.I.H.M.?

- C.I.H.M. exists to promote and develop the authentic therapy through education research.
- To establish and maintain a high professional standard for Indian Head Massage.
- To establish a reputation for excellence through regulation.
- To promote the holistic health benefits of Indian Head Massage to society.
- To facilitate communication amongst those involved in professional practice.

What are the functions of C.I.H.M.?

- Provides professional training courses in Indian Head Massage through The Confederation of Ayurvedic Therapy (C.A.T.).
- Organises conferences, seminars and workshops.
- Produces a member's newsletter (quarterly).
- Members maintain professional standards and are bound by the Confederation's professional code of conduct.

Who can join C.I.H.M.?

- Lecturers of Indian Head Massage.
- Practitioners of Indian Head Massage.
- Students of Indian Head Massage.
- Practitioners of Holistic/Ayurvedic therapies.

Appendix Two

Dr. P. Kulkarni, president of the European Academy of Ayurveda verified the information on Ayurveda. He may be contacted at: Seth Tarachand Hospital, Pune, India. Tel: 91 020 6120296 (hospital); 91 020 6124755 (college).

Jolanta Basnyet, who provided the information on the carrier oils used in Indian Head Massage, holds a degree in Complementary Medicine from the University of Central Lancashire. She is the Principal of the Lancashire Holistic College and proprietor of the Natural Health Centre in Preston. She holds bona fide professional qualifications in the field of Body Massage, Indian Head Massage, Aromatherapy and Reflexology. She is also qualified and fully trained as an osteopath. She is the author of a book on body massage.

Her handmade natural skin and hair care aromatherapy products, prepared in small batches, can be purchased from her retail outlet Jolanta Health Products in Preston or ordered via the internet on www.jolanta.co.uk, or tel: 01772 825177.

The first aid information was provided by: Russell King, 18 Hutchison Drive, Darvel, Ayrshire, KA17 0BL.

Glossary of Terms

Aakasha	Space.
Agada Tantra	Toxicology.
Agni	Fire.
Ajna	The Third Eye Chakra.
Alochaka Pitta	Situated in the eye, its functions are vision and discrimination of colours.
Anahata	The Heart Chakra.
Anna-Vaha	Food passage.
Artava	Menstrual blood.
Asthi	Bone and connective tissues.
Asthi-Vaha	Connective tissue.
Atipravutti	Excessive flow.
Atma	Spirit/soul.
Avalambaka Kapha	Located in the chest and provides nutrition to the heart.
Ayurveda	Science of life.
Bhrajaka Pitta	Provides pigment to the skin, hair.
Bhuta Vidya	Psychotherapy.
Bodhaka Kapha	Found in the tongue and is responsible for perceiving taste.
Brahmand	Tenth gate.
Chakra	Spinning wheel of energy.
Dhatu	Derived from the verb 'Dha' which means 'to hold'. The tissues which hold the body are termed as Dhatu.
Dosha	Differentiate between living and non-living entities.
Dushya	Disease.

Gandha	Odour/smell.
Hrudya	Heart.
Indriya	Senses.
Jala	Water.
Kandara	Tendons.
Kapha	Also called Shleshma. One of its main functions is to provide nutrition to the bodily tissues.
Kaumara Bhrutya	Paediatric and obstetric.
Kayachikitsa	Internal medicine.
Kledaka Kapha	Situated in the stomach. Moistens food and protects the digestive organs from being hurt by the digestive juices.
Kshaya	Decrease.
Majja	Bone marrow.
Majja-Vaha	Bone marrow.
Mala	Different excretions which can be adversely affected with Dhosa imbalances and are often seen as an initial symptom of disease or Dushya where abnormal excretion patterns are observed.
Mala Kapha	Lubricants for joint mobility, digestion and protection from acid attack of internal tissues.
Mala Pitta	Digestive enzyme excretions and natural oils for protection of skin and hair takes place.
Malish	Massage.
Mamsa-Vaha	Muscular tissue.
Mana	Mind.
Manipura	The Solar Plexus Chakra.
Meda	Fatty tissue.
Meda-Vaha	Fat.
Muladhara	The Base Chakra.
Mutra-Vaha	Urinary channels.
Nakha	Nails.
Pancha Mahabhuta	The five basic Universal elements.
Pitta	Derived from the root 'Tapa' which means 'heat' (Santapa).
Pradosha	Vitiation or disabling.

Prana-Vaha	Channels through which oxygen and carbon dioxide exchange.
Pruthvi	Earth.
Purisha-Vaha	Channel for faeces.
Purusha	When Atma (soul) joins with Pancha Mahabhuta (five basic Universal elements) then matter assumes life.
Rajas	Passion.
Rakta	Blood.
Rakta-Vaha	Blood circulation.
Ranjaka Pitta	Liver and spleen. Its main function is to convert Rasa (plasma fluid) into Rakta (blood).
Rasa	Nourishing fluid of plasma.
Rasa-Vaha	Plasma movement.
Rasayana	Rejuvenation.
Rupa	Colour.
Sadhaka Pitta	Located in the Hrudaya (heart) and is responsible for intelligence and ego. It is due to this Pitta that all the functions of the mind and body are co-ordinated.
Sahasrara	The Crown Chakra.
Samadhi	The seat of consciousness, the seat of self and the abode of self in unconscious-conscious state.
Sangraha	Accumulation.
Satva	Mind.
Shabda	Sound.
Shalakya Tantra	Otorhinolaryngology (ENT) and ophthalmology.
Shalya Tantra	Surgery.
Sharira	Body.
Shika	Hair grown in crest/cowlick.
Shira	Vessels.
Shleshaka Kapha	Located in the joints where it provides lubrication.
Shukra	Vital substance.
Shukra-Vaha	Semen.
Sira-Granthi	Thrombosis.
Snayu	Muscle.
Sparsha	Touch.
Srotas	Derived from 'Sru' which means oozing. The oozing of nourishing fluid and the return of waste matters take place through these Srotas.
Stanya	Breast milk.
Swastha	Health.

Swasthavrutta	Healthy.
Sweda	Sweat.
Sweda-Vaha	Channels for sweat.
Svadhistana	The Sacral Chakra.
Tamas	Darkness.
Tarpaka Kapha	Situated in the head and gives nutrition to the mental faculties.
Tikshagni	Extensive.
Twak	Skin.
Udaka-Vaha	Water-balance.
Vajikarana	Aphrodisiac.
Vasa	Fat.
Vata	Derived from the verb 'Va' which means 'to move'.
Vayu	Air.
Vimarga-Gamana	Leakage/haemorrhage.
Vishmagni	Irregular.
Vishudha	The Throat Chakra.
Vruddhi	Increase.

Useful Addresses

The Confederation of Indian Head Massage, including professional courses in Indian Head Massage, can be contacted at: 6 Mayo Crescent, Bankfoot, Bradford, BD5 8JB. Tel: 07703 263132.

Index